GLAUCOMA

What Every Patient
Should Know

Harry A Quigley MD

Table of Contents

*Throughout this guide, the sections above are highlighted in **bold print** to point the reader to those sections that have more detail on the subject covered in them.*

Tell me about you

Foreword

You or a member of your family has been told that you have glaucoma. Or, you have had glaucoma for some time and are concerned that the treatment you're receiving isn't right for you. To help you answer the many questions about this common eye disease, I wrote this guide to give authoritative answers, easily understood explanations, helpful suggestions, and life-style advice. It won't matter if you are not a medical specialist, since the guide is written in plain English. Most glaucoma patients retain good vision and live a normal life. The solutions given here can take the stress out of dealing with glaucoma and should maximize the chance that no further injury to your ability to see will occur.

When someone comes for a glaucoma consultation for the first time, I start by asking: "Tell me about you". I do this because getting to know each other is the most important aspect of a long-term relationship. This relationship is the one which will help you keep your vision for as long as you need it. If you've read this far, you have already taken an important first step in that process. You are showing an interest in knowing more. The purpose of this guide is to provide information that will help us to inform you and provide the facts that you need to deal with this treatable problem.

Believe it or not, on hearing the initial news that they may have glaucoma, many people think things like: "I probably don't really have glaucoma"; or "The diagnosis was wrong"; or, "I never did anything bad to get it, so it can't have happened". When people deny that they really have glaucoma, the sad result is that some of them stop coming for exams and do not follow advice about taking eye drops. Some rely only on "alternative" therapies. Learning about each patient, who they are, what they do, are they a Mom or Dad or a Grandparent, helps doctors to find the best solutions to caring for them as individuals. Some people want detailed scientific explanations and like to see videos of eye surgery. Others need simple solutions and don't want too much detail. Here, you can get both. If you want the highlights, there are "Take Home" messages at the start of each section with the most important information. For those wishing to know much more in any section, the details follow. If you still want more, online Internet links are given and a full online version of this book can be reached at this site: www.hopkinsmedicine/wilmerinstitute/glaucoma.

This guide's sections are designed to answer the many questions that patients have asked me in 40 years of practice, as well as the questions that they *should* have asked. For those who know little about their glaucoma, it begins with a simple introduction to the disease. However, those who want in depth information should not be disappointed. Illustrations assist in understanding concepts, parts of the eye, and surgical treatments. There are not perfect or settled answers to every question about glaucoma. Where there is controversy, I present the different sides of the issue to help you and your doctor to make the better choice for you. Since there is no cure for glaucoma, and no means as yet to restore vision once it is lost, the guide presents ways to continue life at a high level, whatever the stage of glaucoma.

Other books have attempted to succeed at these goals, some written by lay persons and others written by doctors with professional writers. I wrote this guide, with help from my colleagues at the

Glaucoma Center of Excellence, Wilmer Eye Institute, to stick closely to actual interactions I've had working with patients to manage their glaucoma and their lives. Often, patients come with lists of questions or pages printed from Internet sites from which they try to inform themselves. I encourage this knowledge-seeking, because there is good evidence that patients who try to learn more will do better in the long run. But, it is very hard to figure out what to believe, even for medically trained people. I learned this lesson in trying to help a family member with prostate cancer. I'm a University clinician scientist who should be able to evaluate medical questions and determine the best course. Instead, I was humbled by trying to look at the vast literature, the many web sites, and knowing what to believe. The right thing to do was to read the comprehensive Dr. Patrick Walsh's Guide to Surviving Prostate Cancer, written by my Johns Hopkins colleague and internationally known leader in the field. We read Pat's book, then had a consult with Dr. Walsh, and the right course became clear. It is my hope that this guide will fill a similar need for persons with glaucoma.

What is glaucoma?

TAKE HOME POINTS:

- Glaucoma often has no symptoms
- Nerve cells in eye die slowly
- Vision off to the side is affected first
- Once vision is lost it can't be regained
- Glaucoma is related to eye pressure

Most likely, you were told you had or might have glaucoma at a routine exam of your eyes and had no idea that anything might be wrong. Most common types of glaucoma give no indication that they're there (the medical term for this is that the disease is asymptomatic). There are two main types of glaucoma: open angle and angle closure glaucoma. Half of the people in the developed world with these types of glaucoma don't know they have the diseases, while in the developing world most cases are unfortunately undiagnosed and untreated. This is partly because some people don't go for eye exams. It is also because not all eye doctors recognize glaucoma when they examine the eye.

When you look at something, the light strikes the surface of your eyes and a description of what you see is transmitted to your brain. Your eye has several major parts that assist in this job. Each of the parts is made up of cells, the building blocks of your body. These cells have different specialized jobs; some hold your body together like bricks and mortar, while others send messages to each other like a cell phone sending through towers to another cell phone. Cells that send messages (called retinal ganglion cells, because they are found in the part of the eye called the retina) are particularly important in glaucoma because it is these cells that are damaged in the disease. When light comes into the eye, the light is received first in cells called rods and cones. These cells (also called photoreceptors, because they receive the light) send information about what you are seeing to a second layer of cells, and finally layer 2 cells light up layer 3, the ganglion cells.

Ganglion cells are the cells that die in glaucoma. Once they die, they are not replaced by new cells. This is not true in your skin or even on the front surface of the eye, the cornea, both of which make new cells all the time. But ganglion cells are truly a part of your brain even though they are somewhat outside the brain in the eye. There is a good reason why brain nerve cells don't make new ones normally. We must think of how complex the brain is. There are 1 trillion nerve cells in the human brain and each has about 100 connections or synapses to other nerve cells (100 trillion, or 100,000,000,000,000 for those who like zeroes). In addition, ganglion cells in the retina are surrounded by supporting neurons called amacrine cells and other supporting cells called glia. In the eye there are 3 kinds of glia: astroglia, because they are shaped like pointy stars; microglia because they are small; and Müller cells because Dr. Müller got them named for himself. From the time the retina begins to develop in the womb until around the time of birth, nerve cells are turning into the various types that will be present in the adult (about 10 kinds in the retina). And, up until the age of 6 years of age, the eye's nerve cells are still forming their final permanent connections to other nerve cells in the eye and to partner cells in the brain. Some eye nerve cells connect to other nerve cells at both ends, picking up information from a previous layer and passing it along to the next layer. The ganglion cells that die in glaucoma are that kind of double-ended neuron.

Even more amazing, ganglion cells pick up all the information from all the other nerve cells in the retina and carry it out of the eye on their one fiber through the optic nerve head (Figure 1) to the next way-station in the brain (the lateral geniculate). From there, there is another relay to the back of the brain where more complex visual processes go on. The ganglion cell's fiber is amazingly long. If the cell body in the retina were the size of a basketball, the fiber would be as long as a football field (the actual fiber is about 2 inches long). On its way, this fiber has to pass through the wall of the eye to get into the brain. The optic nerve head, where the fiber leaves the eye is the ganglion cell's Achilles heel, a spot where the stress of the eye wall and the need for good blood supply in a tight spot can kink it and disrupt its communication (see section **How did I get glaucoma?**). We have known for a long time that the normal flow of chemicals within the ganglion cell fiber is blocked in glaucoma just where fibers leave the eye, and that this is an important way the ganglion cell is injured and dies.

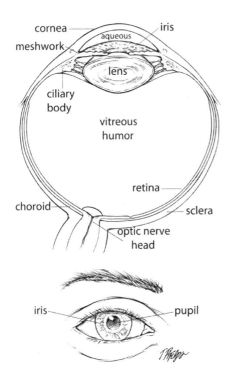

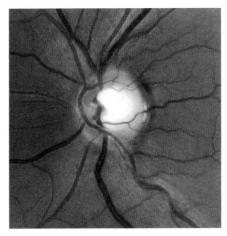

Figure 1: a) The drawings show the main parts of the eye: cornea, iris, lens, trabecular meshwork, ciliary body, aqueous humor, choroid, sclera, retina, and optic nerve head. b) The photograph is the optic nerve head, a round area with blood vessels radiating out from it.

So, once a large number of ganglion cells die from glaucoma, the patient's peripheral vision is affected seriously. How many have to die to really cause vision loss? Glaucoma Center of Excellence research shows that it takes the loss of about 30% of the ganglion cells to reach the point where the doctor's tests (visual field tests) show that the patient's vision is definitely abnormal.

Glaucoma creeps up on us without notice because of several features. First, it involves the slow loss of retinal ganglion cells (Figure 2). Because these cells carry the visual messages through which we see, losing them causes our vision loss. But ganglion cells die so gradually in most glaucoma that we don't notice the loss. We begin life with around one million ganglion cells and barring major eye disease,

75% of them last until we are 90 years old. Glaucoma speeds up the rate at which they die. Each ganglion cell has its own location in the eye to receive light signals over a tiny area that is up to one millimeter wide. Signals travel from the ganglion cells to the brain along a fiber nearly two inches long. As the tiny fibers of each ganglion cell leave the eye, they are vulnerable to being injured at their exit point, the optic nerve head.

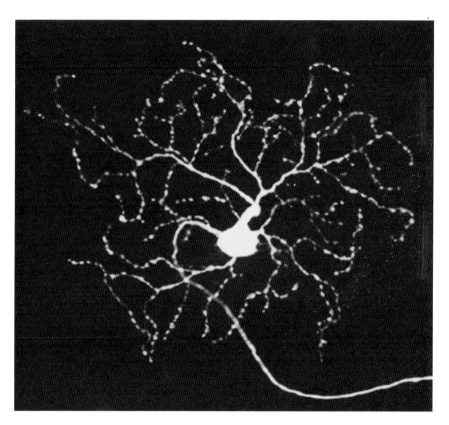

Figure 2: A photograph of a retinal ganglion cell, with its central cell body from which branches spread out to receive messages from other nerve cells. The axon fiber that carries its message out of the eye to the brain leaves the picture at the right. When this fiber passes out of the eye at the optic nerve head, it is injured in glaucoma, causing the ganglion cell to die.

The second reason glaucoma is a silent disease is that the ganglion cells most likely to die are those that provide us with our side vision. Only late in the disease does it attack our center vision, where we have our 20/20 reading ability. We don't rely as much on our side vision as we do the center vision. When we are reading or watching TV or surfing the net, our attention is focused on the object in front of us, not things off to one side. This means that the vision loss from glaucoma is not noticeable in its early stages. You can get a feeling for where the initial damage happens by looking at Figure 3. Close your left eye and hold this book (or computer) at a normal reading distance of about 14 inches. Look at the right page with your right eye, where the words are in **bold print**. The typical place for early glaucoma damage to cause you not to see is on the left page, where some of the print has been removed as an illustration. Since we normally pay most attention to directly where we're reading, most of us would not notice anything wrong if this part of the vision were missing.

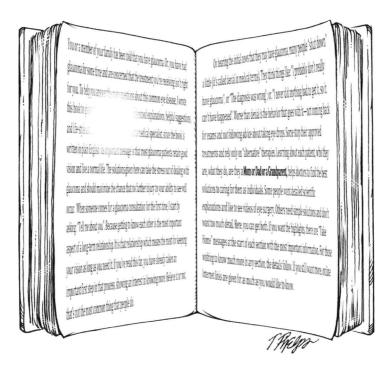

Figure 3: An example of the zone in which early glaucoma vision loss happens. Follow instructions in text for how to view this drawing.

Another reason that glaucoma's damage is not noticed early on is that it typically affects only one eye at first. The other eye is still fully functional. Both eyes get similar information about the world, and the brain converts the two separate signals into a single picture. With both eyes open, as we view the world, any object is seen by both eyes and its image is sent to the brain by both. If the brain gets the image from either eye, we see it and we think nothing is missing. In fact, loss of the image from one eye does cause a loss of the ability to see things in three dimensions. This ability helps us to tell how far away from us something is in space and is called stereoscopic vision. So, we can lose a lot of vision from one eye, but if the other eye is unaffected by glaucoma, we don't notice. Clinical research from our Wilmer Institute Center for Glaucoma Excellence shows that the typical person with glaucoma loses twice as much vision in the worse-affected eye compared to the better eye, but if left untreated, eventually both eyes become abnormal and this really decreases our ability to enjoy life.

Fourth, we're pretty adaptable creatures, and we alter our behavior to take account of the damage, even without knowing it. When investigators evaluate how much glaucoma damage it takes to affect patient's daily activities, they find that damage has to be pretty bad before it is recognized as a problem. Yet, when the actual functional capability is measured, in such things as reading, walking, and driving, it is clear that persons with significant glaucoma damage read more slowly, walk more carefully, bump into things more, and give up driving sooner than others.

One fundamental fact is that vision lost from glaucoma does not come back and no present treatment can restore it. Some parts of your body, such as your skin, can recover from damage because those organs can build new cells to replace damaged cells. This is not true for nerve cells in the brain or the eye. The ganglion cells that are damaged in glaucoma cannot be fixed or replaced once they are damaged. The layer of nerve tissue in the eye that contains the ganglion cells (the retina) is a very complicated network of 10 types of cells. Ganglion cells are the only ones to die from glaucoma, but their loss causes rearrangements in the retina and up in the brain's relay centers to which they go. To put back function, we will need to insert new nerve cells in their place, to reconnect the new cells to the cells that are still there, and to make those connections work with the existing connections in the way that they did originally. While our laboratory, along with others, has taken the first steps in this process, it is a long way to go to successfully restore vision in a human eye (see section **Can glaucoma be cured?** for more details).

One final important fact is that all of the forms of glaucoma are related to some degree to the pressure inside the eye. The eye is something like a camera, with lenses at the front (called the cornea and the lens) and the film or the digital receiving surface at the back (the retina; see Figure 1). For clear vision, we need the image placed on the retina and not moving, since if it is not stable, it would seem blurred. The eye is filled with fluid which must be kept within a narrow range of pressure, like the air pressure inside of a bicycle tire.

The fluid inside the eye is not the fluid we make when our eyes tear (or whey we cry). Tears come from glands outside the eye and are not directly related to glaucoma. Like a bicycle tire, the eye must have the correct pressure inside to work properly. The balance between fluid flowing in and out of the eye maintains a higher pressure inside the eye than outside. This pressure difference produces stress in the eye wall (sclera), keeping it tense and stable so that the retina's image is clear.

The normal eye pressure is about 15 millimeters of mercury. This is enough pressure to make the images stable on the retina by keeping the wall of the eye firm. The wall of the eye is made of 3 layers: the white outer layer or sclera, the middle layer containing blood vessels (the choroid), and the retina with its nerves. Pressure is maintained by having fluid come into the eye at one location (the ciliary body) and leave through the main outflow zone (the trabecular meshwork). The continuous flow of this fluid (the aqueous humor) also nourishes the structures inside the eye that have no blood supply of their own.

Whether the eye pressure is a bit lower or higher, there is always some physical tension (called stress by engineers) in the sclera. The higher the pressure, the more is the stress. Because the fibers of ganglion cells must go through the sclera at the optic nerve head to go up to the brain, they are damaged by this stress (Figure 4).

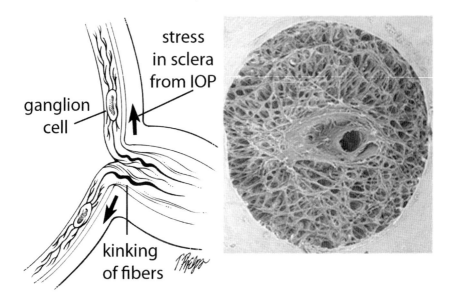

Figure 4: Drawing at the left shows 2 ganglion cells (shaped like spiders) in the retina and their fiber passing to the nerve head. In the nerve head, the fibers are injured by stress (arrows) applied to them or to their supporting tissues, which causes kinking of fibers. At the right, the support structure of the nerve head is seen from inside the eye. Ganglion cell fibers pass out of the eye through the many small holes. Stress in the eye wall pulls on this structure and damages the fibers (which were removed to make this picture).

Ganglion cells are damaged by prolonged eye wall stress and this is the cause of damage to your vision in glaucoma. This means that the higher the pressure, the greater the chance for glaucoma. However, not everyone's eyes react to pressure in the same way. The fibers in some people's eyes can tolerate greater amounts of pressure that others. If my eye has a thinner wall than yours, or is bigger in diameter, it will have more stress from the same amount of pressure (Figure 5).

Think of the eye as a water balloon filled to some pressure. If the balloon has a thick wall, it will be harder to get it to expand than if the wall is thin. In the eye, the balloon wall is the clear cornea and the white sclera. Certain rules of physics say that if two balloons are filled to the same pressure, but one is bigger than the other one, the stress in the balloon wall is larger in the bigger one. The reason the stress in the wall is important is that ganglion cells have to send their fiber out through an opening in the wall, the optic nerve head, to get their message to the brain. The fiber gets hurt by stress in the eye wall as it passes through. It's like the canyon in the western movie, where the hero has to pass between narrow walls and the bad guys ambush him. In the eye, the fibers pass out with some tissue supporting the opening, called the lamina cribrosa (Figure 5). That structure is most like a colander that we use to drain spaghetti, the fibers of ganglion cells go out the holes and the struts around the holes try to resist the stress put on them by the wall of the eye pulling outward. The struts also have to resist the pressing from inside out, since the pressure inside the eye is higher than outside.

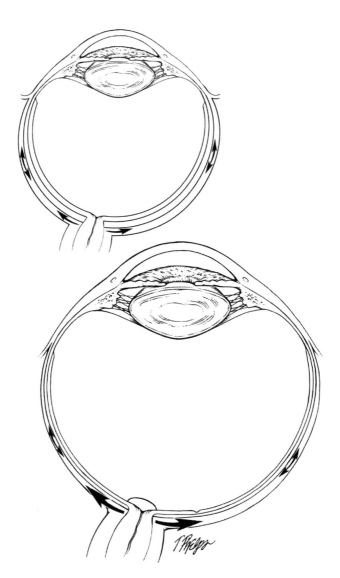

Figure 5: Drawings show small eye with thicker eye wall (above) and larger eye with thinner wall (below). There is stress in the eye wall from eye pressure in both eyes (arrows), but the stress is greater (bigger arrows) in the big, thin-walled eye. Near-sighted (myopic) eyes are therefore more likely to get open angle glaucoma.

So, glaucoma can happen at any pressure, as long as the effects of stress are sufficient to kill ganglion cells. In fact, half of those with the most common type of glaucoma, called open angle glaucoma, always have a normal level of eye pressure. In their eyes, the stress of normal pressure (combined with other features) is enough to kill ganglion cells. Therefore, it is not necessarily "elevated" pressure that is the enemy in glaucoma (see **Low tension glaucoma doesn't exist**). All present treatment for glaucoma is designed reduce the damaging level of pressure found in the untreated person, lowering it to a safer level that will allow no further damage (see **What is the target pressure?**).

Experts say that glaucoma has started as a definite disease in a person when one of the eyes has suffered actual structural and functional damage. This damage shows up as specific abnormalities on standard examination tests (see **What tests are needed to diagnose glaucoma?**). Before this point, there are many persons who are suspected to have glaucoma but have not met the official damage criteria, and they are called glaucoma suspects. In the offices of many eye doctors, these strict definitions are not obeyed—some doctors use the term glaucoma more broadly to mean anyone whom they intend to treat.

The next sections describe the various types of glaucoma and how they differ.

What are the types of glaucoma?

> **TAKE HOME POINTS:**
>
> - Four types of glaucoma: open angle, angle closure, secondary, childhood
> - Open angle glaucoma is not divided into lower and higher pressure types
> - Acute angle closure attack is an emergency
> - Angle closure treatment starts with laser iridotomy
> - Glaucoma can happen due to another eye condition (secondary)
> - Children can have glaucoma as early as the first year of life

There are 60 million persons in the world with some form of glaucoma. This estimate is based on surveys that examined thousands of randomly selected adults in nearly every continent. At our Glaucoma Center of Excellence, researchers project that by the year 2020 there will be 80 million people with glaucoma around the world, 20 million more than in 2010. This increase will be due to that fact that the proportion of older people in the world population is increasing compared to young people, and glaucoma is more likely to occur in older people. Glaucoma is the second leading cause of blindness worldwide.

WHAT ARE THE TYPES OF GLAUCOMA?

There are several forms of glaucoma, and the two most common forms increase with older age. At 40 years old, less than one in 100 persons have glaucoma, while over age 80, nearly one in ten is affected. These rates are different depending upon ethnic derivation and other factors. For example, African-Americans have four times more open angle glaucoma than persons who are European-derived. For angle closure glaucoma, Asians have four times more than either European- or African-derived persons.

Of those with glaucoma, the majority (about two-thirds) have the form called open angle glaucoma. In the United States alone, there are estimated to be 2.25 million adults with open angle glaucoma, about 500,000 with angle closure glaucoma, and another 5-10 million persons who are potential glaucoma patients (glaucoma suspects) due to various kinds of risk factors. Risk factors are features of their eyes or other attributes that make glaucoma more likely to develop.

Both major types of glaucoma have the word "angle" in their name. The angle is a circular zone on the inside part of the eye where the cornea, the clear front wall of the eye, meets the iris, the blue or brown part of the eye. This angle area runs all around the part of the eye where the white sclera and the colored iris meet. In general, an individual either has an open angle or a narrow to closed angle (Figure 6). This is determined by the examination called gonioscopy (see **What tests are needed to diagnose glaucoma?**).

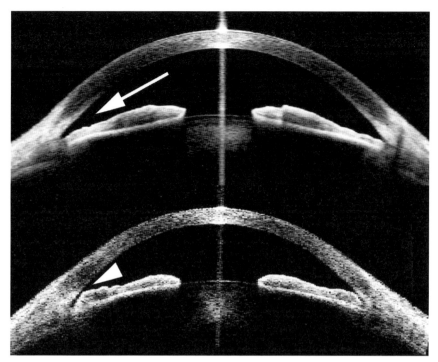

Figure 6: A slice through the front of two eyes taken with a special camera shows an open angle above and a closed angle below (images made with anterior segment optical coherence tomography). The arrow points to where the iris is separate from the cornea in the open angle (upper picture). In the lower picture, the iris is so close to the cornea that it nearly touches the trabecular meshwork (in front of arrowhead).

The aqueous humor fluid nourishes the eye, circulates from back to front, and maintains the eye pressure. Fluid normally moves from where it is produced, the ciliary body, between the lens and the back of the iris, through the round, black opening in the iris called the pupil and leaves the eye at the trabecular meshwork in the angle. Just at the base of the meshwork, fluid can also move out through a second pathway called the uveoscleral outflow. In most eyes, fluid gets to the angle from the back of the eye easily, and these are open angle eyes. In a few eyes, the parts of the eye in the front are too crowded together, and the colored iris can get close enough to block the angle at the meshwork. These are angle closure eyes.

Open Angle Glaucoma

By numbers alone, the majority of those with glaucoma have the open angle type. In the eyes with open angle glaucoma, the structures that make aqueous humor and the outflow channels are normal in appearance when the doctor examines them. Those eyes with diseased outflow channels have problems at the microscopic level. Open angle glaucoma can happen at any level of eye pressure, and half of those with open angle glaucoma have normal levels of eye pressure. This often surprises those who think of glaucoma as always due to high eye pressure. Glaucoma can occur at normal levels of eye pressure due to weaknesses in the eye that kill ganglion cells. Some of these weaknesses have been identified at the microscopic, genetic and biochemical levels. We will deal with these in more detail in the next section **How did you get glaucoma?**

For the other half of those with open angle glaucoma, the pressure that damages their vision is actually above normal. In these persons, various abnormalities lead the eye pressure to be high, and, if the eye and ganglion cells are susceptible to the effects of such higher pressure, glaucoma ensues. There are different theories for why the eye pressure is above normal in open angle glaucoma eyes with higher pressure. The best explanation is that there is a problem that prevents fluid from leaving the eye correctly within the angle. The most likely reason for this is premature death of the cells in the aqueous outflow area of the angle. Another probable factor is blockage of the outflow channels by very tiny collections of material that shouldn't be there. Because the primary cause of disease in this group of open angle glaucoma patients is poor flow through the meshwork, some new potential treatments for open angle glaucoma try to improve this flow. Since lowering eye pressure helps all persons with glaucoma, this could help both those with the higher and the lower pressure types of open angle glaucoma.

Angle Closure Glaucoma

Normally, aqueous humor fluid moves from the back chamber of the eye into the front chamber of the eye, after which it goes back into the blood stream. To move from back to front, it must pass between the iris and the lens and through the pupil opening (Figure 7). Angle closure eyes are generally smaller in all dimensions than average. The passageway is very narrow in smaller eyes and the fluid can get blocked in trying to move through. This is known as pupil block. In angle closure glaucoma, the iris is so close to the trabecular meshwork that when pupil block increases, it pushes the iris against the meshwork, blocking the outflow of aqueous humor. The lens in angle closure eyes is also more forward (meaning it is closer to the cornea), increasing the difficulty for aqueous humor to pass between the lens and iris on its way to the anterior chamber. When this resistance is very high (more pupil block), the pressure behind the iris is greater than in front of it, making the iris billow forward like a sail in a strong breeze. If this forward iris movement carries it to the point of closing the angle, drainage is blocked and eye pressure rises.

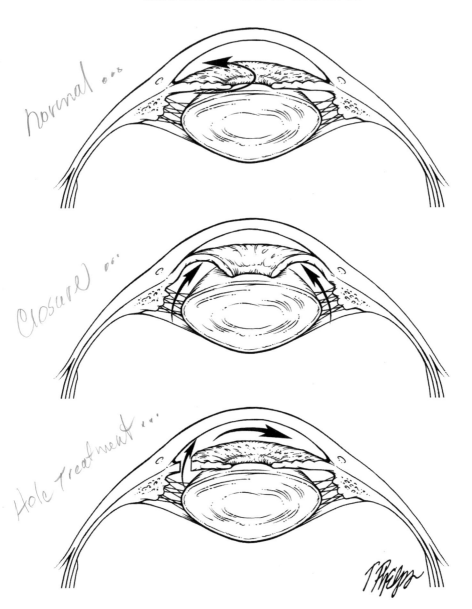

Figure 7: Aqueous humor normally passes from behind the iris to in front of the iris through the pupil (arrow in upper drawing). In angle closure, aqueous is trapped behind the iris, causing the iris to bow forward and block the outflow of aqueous humor (middle drawing). The initial treatment for angle closure is to make a hole in the iris with laser to prevent pupil block and iris bowing (bottom drawing).

The increase in eye pressure in angle closure eyes can be intermittent and moderate, or less commonly, sudden and drastic. This sudden increase is called an acute angle closure crisis or attack. The **Acute angle closure crisis** (see that section) is actually uncommon, happening only in a minority of all those with angle closure. It can lead to severe, permanent vision damage in days if not treated promptly, and other consequences of angle closure are more severe in those with this acute crisis. People who have an acute crisis can rapidly develop haziness in the lens (a condition called cataract) and frequently need glaucoma surgery to resolve elevation of eye pressure (see **Operations for glaucoma**).

Typical symptoms of the acute angle closure crisis are eye pain, nausea, headaches, halos around lights, and severely blurred vision. The pupil increases in size in response to low light levels or drugs which artificially increase its size, called dilation. Sudden acute angle closure attacks are more likely to occur when the pupil is partially dilated, for example, being in a darkened room such as a movie theater, or when pills or eye drops are taken that dilate the pupil. This can happen to persons at risk for angle closure when they have a standard eye exam, in which dilation of the pupil is done to examine the inside of the eye. Acute angle-closure crisis is a true emergency, for which immediate eye exam and treatment are vision-saving. Emergency room medical personnel should always check eye pressure in persons with severe headache, since acute attacks can be so severe that the whole head hurts. The pain makes some persons nauseated and their vomiting is occasionally misinterpreted as an acute abdominal problem.

A number of medications can initiate acute angle closure crisis by dilating the pupil, including cold tablets and pills taken for incontinence. The FDA marks these as potentially dangerous for those with "glaucoma," but fails to mention that this is only true for persons with angle closure (not those with open angle glaucoma). After the initial treatment, making a hole in the iris by laser iridotomy, the blockage of aqueous humor no longer occurs and angle closure patients can take these types of medications without risk.

Based on research conducted by Glaucoma Center of Excellence researchers at Johns Hopkins, there are a number of other features of the eye's behavior that contribute to angle closure and angle closure glaucoma. These are considered in the next section (see **How did you get glaucoma?**). However, it is a good idea to make a laser hole in the iris for several groups:

- Those with signs that the angle is critically narrow
- Those that have an acute angle closure crisis
- Those in whom the angle closure has caused glaucoma (structural and functional damage to the ganglion cells and optic nerve head)

Description of laser iridotomy, the initial angle closure treatment is presented in **Laser glaucoma surgery: iris holes and angle treatment**.

Secondary Glaucoma

Typical open angle and angle closure glaucoma are called primary glaucoma, since they are diseases in and of themselves. Glaucoma can also be a result of other eye conditions or general body diseases. This is referred to as secondary glaucoma because it is caused by "something else" (see section on **Secondary glaucoma**). In secondary glaucoma, the damage always comes from having an eye pressure higher than the normal range. In nearly every case, the reason for the abnormally high pressure is some obstruction to outflow of aqueous humor through the trabecular meshwork.

One of the most common kinds of secondary glaucoma happens when new blood vessels grow in the eye and block aqueous outflow (neovascular glaucoma). This can happen in patients who have had diabetes mellitus for some years. It also happens when blood flow to the eye is disturbed by obstruction of the main vein that drains the retina inside the eye (central vein occlusion) or by obstruction in the large arteries that connect the heart to the brain and eye (carotid artery occlusion). There are specific diagnostic tests for blood flow in the eye called fluorescein angiography and also there are non-invasive tests for flow in the carotid arteries using ultrasound machines. In cases of neovascular glaucoma related to diabetes and central vein occlusion, specific laser treatment of the retina is performed to eliminate these new blood vessels (pan-retinal photocoagulation). More recently, retinal specialists have added injections into the eye of anti-blood vessel medicines (blockers of vascular endothelial growth factor). This is done under local anesthesia in the office.

Another common form of secondary glaucoma occurs when corticosteroid drugs are taken, leading to higher than normal eye pressure. There are many different chemical names for "steroids" of this type, with the most common name being prednisone or cortisone. These agents are given as pills, nasal sprays, inhalers, and by injection into joints and even into the eye for some conditions. We formerly thought that one had to have a special gene to be a "steroid responder", but we now recognize that a high enough dose delivered to the eye itself can cause eye pressure increase in nearly everyone. So, it is more a matter of degree of risk than an all or none response. While there is a "glaucoma caution" on the Food and Drug Administration paperwork for all such drugs, many non-eye doctors and patients using these agents do not know you have glaucoma. Among the common disorders for which steroids are given are asthma and arthritis—but the steroid can be mixed in with other drugs in combination and the name may not be a good clue. When eye pressure rises due to corticosteroids, it can be lowered by typical glaucoma medications or even surgery. Removal of delivered steroid or stopping the medicine will also help to normalize the eye pressure. Naturally, those who already have glaucoma are at more risk from such an increase in pressure than are those with no existing glaucoma. Patients who are given "eye drops" from non-eye physicians may not be aware that these are often combinations of antibiotics and corticosteroids, and that the regular use of such eye drops can over an extended period lead to vision loss.

Those who undergo eye surgery for conditions other than glaucoma can have an eye pressure that becomes and stays high; this is considered glaucoma secondary to surgery. The operation to treat cataract is generally successful and uncomplicated, but a small number of patients will have complications including high eye pressure. Or, secondary glaucoma can be a result of another major eye disease that leads to blocking of aqueous humor outflow. Since eye pressure is nearly always measured by eye doctors who are taking care of these eyes, the situation rarely goes unnoticed. Medical and surgical glaucoma treatment may need to be added to the already performed procedures.

Severe injuries to the eye can cause traumatic glaucoma, due either to damage to the trabecular meshwork by the blow or rupture of the eye wall, or by blood in the eye and other obstructive material blocking the outflow of aqueous. Many of these secondary, injury-related glaucoma situations are temporary and quiet down without need for long-term treatment. Some, however, become threats to vision and require long term treatment.

Various conditions cause inflammation in the eye and increase eye pressure (inflammatory glaucoma). In each part of our body, defense mechanisms ward off invading bacteria and viruses or respond to injury in their own way. When we get a cold or flu our nose runs, we cough, and the skin can get red and itchy from blood vessel reactions. These are all natural ways our body fights off the infection and returns us to health, but they feel unpleasant while they happen. Inflammatory diseases happen when the normal defense reactions get activated incorrectly, and actually cause disease by themselves. In the eye, this happens with forms of arthritis, with cancers like lymphoma, with HIV-AIDS, and sometimes for no known reason (in this case the disease is called "idiopathic"). Inflammation blocks up outflow of aqueous and so causes secondary glaucoma. Anti-inflammatory medicines include corticosteroids, which as mentioned already can raise the pressure further if the inflammation isn't stopped promptly. So inflammatory glaucoma can respond to standard glaucoma therapy, but is sometimes very tough to treat.

Childhood Glaucoma

While glaucoma in infants and children happens only once in several thousand births, it is vitally important for new parents and pediatricians to be aware of its signs and symptoms. We have devoted an entire section to this subject (**Childhood glaucoma**). This is because the diagnosis and treatment of glaucoma in kids are different in many ways from adults.

How did you get glaucoma?

TAKE HOME POINTS:

- **You did not do anything wrong to cause it**
- **There is more than one "cause" for glaucoma**
- **In general, your personal habits, diet, and exposure to the world don't cause glaucoma**
- **Features called risk factors for open angle and angle closure glaucoma are somewhat different**
- **Stress in the eye wall damages nerve fibers as they leave the eye, even at normal eye pressure**

Common factors in open angle and angle closure glaucoma

In this section, we'll talk about the causes of two main types of primary glaucoma, open angle and angle closure. The things that are known to cause each of these two disorders are a bit different. But, the damage in both of them happens in the same general way after they get started, and many of the treatments are similar. For any complicated disease like glaucoma, there are no easy answers. It doesn't come from only one thing or a single abnormality. To speak of one cause of a disease is simply not possible. The eye has many interconnecting parts, and each cell that makes up those parts is almost infinitely complex in the interweaving electrical and chemical pathways that help the cell to survive. And, as we will see, there are equally intricate pathways that tell the nerve cells to kill themselves under conditions where the disease is active. (Yes, they actually commit suicide).

One of the first questions we are often asked is: "what did I do that caused glaucoma?" To a large degree, the answer is "nothing"—there are almost no life-style choices that are known to be big factors in leading to either form of glaucoma. We will talk about personal behaviors that can help a bit with your glaucoma in the section **How should you change your life?** For example, we know that cigarette smoking and over-exposure to sunshine can be big contributors to two other eye diseases in older persons—cataract and age-related macular degeneration. But, smoking and sunlight are not at all related to glaucoma. Instead, it seems the most important things that determine glaucoma risk are how the eye was built and how it responds to changes in its environment.

The death of ganglion cells in both open angle and angle closure glaucoma results partly from weaknesses in the tissues around them and partly from defects in the ganglion cells themselves. It also results from under-responses or over-responses in our normal defense mechanisms. These factors can gang up to produce glaucoma by having several things go wrong at the same time. In fact, glaucoma probably happens only when more than one process is malfunctioning. Each of the single things that are part of the disease package is called a contributing risk factor. Together, all the contributing factors that wind up causing the glaucoma make up sufficient cause for it to occur. The mixed bag of contributors to the sufficient cause can be different among people—even among members of the same family each of whom has glaucoma.

One major cause of the death of ganglion cells in both major types of primary glaucoma is how the wall of the eye responds to eye pressure. We showed earlier how it can be worse in glaucoma to have a big, thin-walled eye than a smaller one, since the stress in the eye wall is higher (Figure 5). The fibers of ganglion cells get injured when the eye wall stress affects the optic nerve head and presses on the fibers passing through it. Not just the nerve fibers

28

are hurt going through the nerve head. Nerve fibers are supported by other kinds of cells and tissues, including the small blood vessels that nourish the fibers at this site. Eye wall stress also affects these cells badly. So the behavior of the eye wall is translated into vision loss by physical stress at a critical place. Eyes that are bigger have more stress, explaining why very near-sighted people with longer eyes get more open angle glaucoma. Even normal-sized eyes whose wall responds badly to stress can kill fibers – in them it happens at eye pressures that most of us tolerate with no damage. This is one explanation for how persons with normal eye pressure can get open angle glaucoma; their eye wall delivers more stress to the nerve fibers at normal pressure than most persons. The critical tissues in the nerve head called the lamina cribrosa probably stand up to the eye wall stress better in some of us and worse in others—causing more glaucoma damage when the lamina is weaker. In persons with angle closure glaucoma, the eye is smaller, which ought to be protective from wall stress, but their eye pressures are typically higher than normal and that produces enough stress to damage fibers and their supporting cells. *"a mixed bag"...*

A lot of other factors are known to contribute to ganglion cell death and therefore to cause glaucoma's vision loss. We know this by studying human eyes of persons who had glaucoma and who donated their eyes after their death to an eye bank. We are often asked by glaucoma patients if it is worthwhile for them to be an eye donor. After all, their eyes are damaged, so surely they aren't useful. Most donated eyes are used to transplant the clear cornea to someone who needs a new one. Eyes from people with glaucoma are not useful for that kind of transplant, but donated glaucoma eyes are vitally important to study how glaucoma does its damage. Many studies have also been conducted with animals in whom glaucoma develops spontaneously or in whom a glaucoma-like condition is produced in one eye.

From the human glaucoma eyes and animal research, we have learned that glaucoma causes harmful chemicals to be released by cells at the optic nerve head and in the retina, where the ganglion cell body lives. The blood nourishing ganglion cells and their fibers

can fail to provide enough oxygen or the energy producing com-
pounds that drive normal processes. We will come back to more of
these contributing features to ganglion cell death in the section **Are
there treatments other than lowering eye pressure?**

We'll now consider the contributing risk factors for open angle
glaucoma and angle closure glaucoma separately from each other,
since in many ways they are different.

Things that make open angle glaucoma more likely
- **Older age**
- **Higher eye pressure (even if it is in the normal range)**
- **Family background (ethnicity)—more common in African, Hispanic**
- **Having blood relatives with it**
- **Being near-sighted (myopic)**
- **Having lower blood pressure (but not high blood pressure)**
- **Having conditions called exfoliation and pigment dispersion**

Other than senior discounts, there are few advantages of getting
older and one of the many disadvantages is a greater chance of
glaucoma (of all types). While open angle glaucoma sometimes
occurs early in life, by far most examples happen after age 60 and
the number affected increases at an increasing rate with older age.
By age 90, nearly one in ten persons has it. Scientists have lots of
suspicions about the many reasons older age would make glaucoma
more likely, but it's obvious that humans systems are more likely to
fail with every passing decade.

The higher the eye pressure, the greater the chance for open
angle glaucoma. About half of cases occur in persons whose eye
pressure without treatment is higher than the normal range. Their
tendency to get glaucoma probably comes from abnormal outflow
of the aqueous humor in the front of the eye. Since water can't
get out fast enough, pressure is not only higher than normal, but
it fluctuates up and down more than in non-glaucoma persons.

HOW DID YOU GET GLAUCOMA?

Both a higher average pressure and a pressure that varies more are factors known to contribute to open angle glaucoma. Millions of persons have eye pressure higher than normal and never develop open angle glaucoma. They are called ocular hypertensives and we discuss them in the section **Why isn't glaucoma either there or not there**—what makes you an open angle glaucoma suspect? Many ocular hypertensive glaucoma suspects fortunately lack some of the other contributing risk factors for open angle glaucoma, or their eyes possess better defense mechanisms against the stress induced by elevated eye pressure. They stay suspects and never get glaucoma. Meanwhile, about half of those with open angle glaucoma never have eye pressure above normal. This situation was once called "low tension" or "normal tension" glaucoma (see section **Low tension glaucoma doesn't exist and you don't have a brain tumor**). Probably their eye wall delivers more stress to the optic nerve head than other eyes at normal eye pressure. This causes death of ganglion cells at eye pressures that most persons have their whole lives without damage. Fortunately, lowering eye pressure is beneficial even in these normal pressure glaucoma patients.

When you have several known contributing risk factors for open angle glaucoma, the collection of factors can be more serious together than they would be individually. For example, among those with a tendency toward glaucoma, it is bad to have low blood pressure and bad to have higher eye pressure—and doubly bad to have the two together. For blood to nourish the optic nerve head and retina, it has to get to the eye, and with low blood pressure coming in and higher eye pressure keeping the blood out, the perfusion pressure is too low. One has to have pretty low blood pressure (or very high eye pressure) to get into a danger zone here, but specialists now keep better track of both blood pressure and eye pressure along with the general doctors who care for open angle glaucoma patients. While blood pressure that is too low may be harmful in glaucoma, we still recommend that high blood pressure be controlled as needed to protect your overall health. Care should be taken not to over treat high blood pressure in persons with glaucoma.

31

Being athletic → ↓ Sym.
Nose Sprays ... allergy Sym. No
• Nose Sprays   Coffee ...

The lower the eye pressure, the better for open angle glaucoma. Some things that make it lower are aerobic exercise, avoidance of corticosteroid medications (even inhaled or nose sprays with steroid), and avoidance of drinking many caffeine-containing drinks per day (see section **How should you change your life**?).

Where your family came from in the world also affects the chance for open angle glaucoma. We now recognize that there is no clear way to test the genes of a person and to properly label them as derived from Africa or Asia or Europe. What is often called "race" is a very complex set of features and the census bureau and scientists studying disease resort to asking someone to state what they call themselves—so-called self-described ethnicity. When you look at the whole population together, we are becoming more related to one another as the world's communication, immigration, and intermarriage increase. Yet, interestingly, when we do a study of how many people have open angle glaucoma and we compare those who self-describe as African-derived (black) and European-derived (white), the rate of glaucoma is 3-4 times higher in the African-derived. The rate of open angle glaucoma is nearly identical for African-derived Baltimore City residents and villagers in central Tanzania in Africa. This seems to tell us that tendency to open angle glaucoma is inherited in a way that doesn't depend heavily on diet, environment, daily or cultural activities, since these things are so different between these two populations of African-derived people. These two groups must share some inherited genetic similarities (see section **Special Section for African-derived persons**). The studies of Hispanic persons also show a higher rate of open angle glaucoma. While we must assume that this is a real worry for this group, the question is even muddier as to whether Hispanics are as homogenous in genetic inheritance terms as other ethnicities. After all, in some studies, people were included as Hispanic because of the language spoken, not their family derivation. We have a colleague who was born in Central America and speaks Spanish as his primary language; he would be Hispanic if studied in Mexico City, yet both his parents came from Central Europe, and if they hadn't moved, he would be classed as European-derived in a study done in Austria. This issue is complicated, indeed!

Many diseases, including glaucoma and breast cancer, can occur more frequently in certain families. These unlucky families have an unusual version of a particular gene that is passed from parents to children and greatly increases the risk of getting the disease. Our genes contribute to open angle glaucoma, and having a close family member affected increases the chance of getting it by 10 times. So, among European-derived adults over age 40, the rate of open angle glaucoma is 2 in 100. But your chance increases to 20 in 100 if your Mom or Dad, brother or sister, or your adult child had or has glaucoma. We often hear "but, no one in my family ever had glaucoma— so why do I have it if it's inherited?" Even though some families have increased risk for glaucoma, people with no family history also get it. Genes aren't the only reason people get glaucoma. Or, perhaps the reason "no one in the family had it" is that they were never examined, or they died prior to getting it, or they didn't tell anyone else in the family that they had it (see section **How can you help your family avoid glaucoma damage?**).

Those with family members who have glaucoma still have a very good chance of NOT getting glaucoma (80%), but, they should be examined regularly, because otherwise they won't know that they have it until it has done serious damage. Routine eye exams can help to avoid unnecessary vision loss in family members who are at risk. On the other side of the coin, we frequently hear from patients that their Mom had glaucoma, only to find out when records of Mom's care are produced that she had cataract, or used daily eye drops for another problem, like dry eyes. In one study, more than half of those who said that they have glaucoma, in fact did not have it—and this was a study of nurses! It is even more important to have regular eye exams for glaucoma if your family member not only had it, but lost vision from it. The tendency to have worse glaucoma is probably inherited, too. At this time, there are 3 known genes in our human DNA that have mistakes called mutations which increase the chance of open angle glaucoma. These make up only a small fraction of all those with glaucoma and at present there is not a good reason to do testing for gene defects as a method to screen for who is going to develop it.

In the section **How did you get glaucoma?** , we explained that people with near-sightedness (myopia) are more likely to get open angle glaucoma. Myopia means you need glasses to see well at distances like 20 feet, but see things held close to your face fairly well without glasses. Myopic eyes are more often longer and have thinner walls. Both features make the stress from any eye pressure worse in causing glaucoma damage. Having laser treatments to change the need for glasses doesn't improve this risk, and those considering such refractive surgery should have careful discussions with the surgeon before doing so for two reasons. First, some forms of refractive surgery use an instrument that raises the eye pressure very high for some minutes. This could theoretically be dangerous for the glaucoma patient. Second, performing these refractive procedures changes the measurement of the eye pressure, typically making it seem lower than it is. We can correct for this best by knowing what pressure was just before and just after the laser refractive procedure. The bottom line is that those who have worn glasses since teen age for myopia should have annual evaluations for glaucoma in adulthood.

Two conditions that make open angle glaucoma more likely are exfoliation syndrome (also called pseudoexfoliation syndrome) and pigment dispersion syndrome (Figure 8). Exfoliation eyes produce a white-dandruff like material that can only be seen inside the front of the eye on the iris and lens. This material is produced by many cells in the body, but mostly causes trouble in the eye. Part of its damage comes from the exfoliation material blocking up the outflow of aqueous humor, so that the eye pressure is both higher and more variable than normal. Both higher pressure and more variable pressure are bad for eyes at risk for glaucoma. Second, there is some evidence that exfoliation eyes are more susceptible to glaucoma because either the structure of the eye or its blood vessels are weaker in exfoliation. We can see exfoliation in detailed eye exams in many persons who don't yet show damage from glaucoma. They are best advised to have more frequent exams than others with less glaucoma risk.

The second internal eye condition that makes open angle glaucoma more likely is pigment dispersion syndrome, which happens in some myopic eyes. Their iris rubs on the structures just behind the iris, the supporting fibers that attach the lens to the eye. Pigment rubs off the back of the iris and blocks the outflow of aqueous humor when the pigment is carried to the trabecular meshwork. Eye doctors can see the places where pigment has rubbed off and the places it deposits on the inner eye, so before there is glaucoma damage it is possible to begin monitoring those with this condition more closely. While exfoliation is more commonly seen in the typical older glaucoma patient, pigment dispersion can begin to cause glaucoma in the 20s and 30s. The features that make pigment dispersion more likely are having a larger eye (being near-sighted) and having an iris that is less in its overall volume. At present, there is controversy about whether making a hole in the iris keeps the pigment from rubbing off in pigment dispersion. If it did, then laser iridotomy treatment would be helpful. A recent controlled clinical study found no benefit of iridotomy for pigment dispersion eyes.

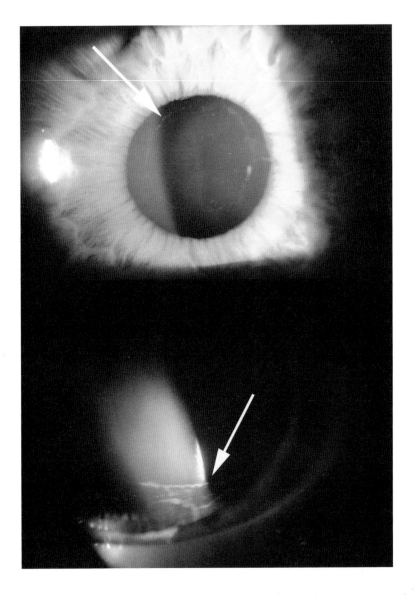

Figure 8: Photograph of an eye with exfoliation syndrome (top) showing white material (arrow) deposited on the lens. Photograph of an eye with pigment dispersion syndrome (bottom) showing excess pigment (arrow) deposited on the area surrounding the lens.

Controversial risk factors for open angle glaucoma

- **Corneal thickness**
- **Heart disease**
- **Anti-cardiolipin**
- **Migraine**
- **Raynaud's phenomenon**

A recent study found that when the thickness of the cornea is measured by a test called pachymetry those with thinner corneas are more likely to go from suspect status to having evidence of open angle glaucoma damage. When we measure eye pressure, the instrument doing the measurement, the tonometer, pushes against the cornea. The higher the eye pressure, the harder it pushes back against the tonometer, giving a higher pressure reading. If the cornea is thin, the instrument will think that the pressure is lower than it really is because it is easier to flatten. So, part of the reason why eyes with thin corneas were more likely to develop glaucoma was that their eye pressure was really higher than the measured number. There is some controversy about whether eyes with thin corneas are more prone to glaucoma even after we take account of the falsely low pressure that is measured. It would make sense that such eyes would be more at risk if having a thin cornea meant that the eye wall all over was thin or that the optic nerve head was more susceptible to pressure. However, this hasn't been shown to be the case (yet).

For many years, it was said that persons with various kinds of heart disease and blood vessel abnormalities were more likely to get glaucoma or to have worse glaucoma when they get it. This is logical, since as we already mentioned, having a low perfusion of blood into the eye (low blood pressure combined with higher eye pressure) is a contributing risk. But, some very extensive studies actually have failed to show that many aspects of cardiovascular disease make glaucoma more likely. This includes things like having had a heart attack, having migraine headaches, and having a constriction of blood vessels in the hands called Raynaud's phenomenon. It may well be that small numbers of persons do have vascular disorders that make glaucoma worse. For example, a recent study found that glaucoma got worse much faster in people who have something in their blood stream called anti-cardiolipin antibodies. But, less than 5 in 100 glaucoma patients had these antibodies.

Things that aren't risk factors for open angle glaucoma
- **Sex (biological gender)**
- **Diabetes**
- **Hypertension**
- **Diet**
- **Alcohol**

People are not "Groups" ... they are individuals with particular Life styles

Men and women get open angle glaucoma at about the same rate. To determine such things, it is important that research studies look at the whole population by some random sampling, as is done in voter's polls before elections where a representative sample is questioned. Otherwise, persons who are more likely to go to the doctor will be found to have a disease more often and it will be incorrectly assumed that they have it more. Women tend to go to doctors in the United States more than men, and women live longer. So doctors who do such studies adjust their estimates by doing random sampling, and by taking account of how many persons at a certain age have the disease. This is called age-specific rates or prevalence.

Some of the most surprising findings about contributing factors to open angle glaucoma have come from recent studies on diabetes mellitus. For years, textbooks taught that diabetes made glaucoma more likely. To be sure, diabetes is a major cause of vision loss, especially when proper diet and exercise recommendations are not followed. But, against the prevailing ideas, more and more studies are showing that having diabetes does not make you more likely to get open angle glaucoma.

Just like diabetes, all the experts formerly said that having high blood pressure was associated with more glaucoma. And, as large studies that examined the question were done, this link became so weak that most studies show no relation at all. In part, it depends on how the study is done. Studies in which glaucoma is defined by having only high eye pressure tend to find that hypertension is related to glaucoma. The more modern open angle glaucoma definition recognizes that eye pressure can be high or low in untreated open angle glaucoma. When this definition is used, there is no contribution of hypertension to open angle glaucoma. There is clearly some link between the level of blood pressure and the level of eye pressure, as the Glaucoma Center of Excellence investigators showed in a large study of healthy adults. They go up or down together to some degree because the systems that control both pressures are similar parts of our unconscious nervous system. Get stressed and both blood and eye pressures tend to rise. Again, it would be foolish to allow yourself to have uncontrolled blood pressure, since that raises the risk of heart attack, stroke and kidney disease.

From a glaucoma viewpoint, there are no dietary or drinking habits that increase the risk of the disease. Drinking a bottle of water very quickly does raise eye pressure, so we recommend you drink slowly to avoid this. Eating a diet with lots of fruits and vegetables is a good health habit. Many studies show that drinking alcohol and caffeine in moderation does not make glaucoma more likely. No nutriceuticals (herbs and the like) have been shown in any decent study to improve the risk of glaucoma (see **Are there treatments other than lowering eye pressure?**). That doesn't mean that you can eat, drink, and be merry, since if you do, you won't live long enough to get glaucoma.

Factors increasing the risk for angle closure glaucoma
- **Older age (again)**
- **Female sex (that's different)**
- **Being Asian**
- **Having blood relatives with it**
- **Having smaller eyes (far-sightedness)**
- **Features of how internal eye structures behave (iris, choroid)**

As with open angle glaucoma, older persons are more likely to have angle closure. We have seen people in their twenties with the disease, but that is very rare. The rate peaks around age 60 or so, at least in part because the natural tendency is for eyes to get shorter (slightly smaller) with time. By contrast with open angle glaucoma, angle closure affects women probably 50% more often than men. The reasons for this aren't completely settled, but we do know that women have smaller eyes and that is one of the contributors.

For reasons that aren't yet fully understood, Asian persons have a lot more angle closure than everyone else in the world, though it may be that east Indians also have a greater risk. Asians don't have more of the other risk factors; at least present research says that their eyes don't have more of the other contributing factors, such as more persons with smaller eyes. Asian eyes look a little different from Europeans because they have different eyelid structure, not because their eyes themselves are a different size. The contribution of family history (genetics) to angle closure is real, but not as well studied as for open angle glaucoma. No actual mutations or DNA code mistakes in particular genes are known that are associated with angle closure yet. Without question, however, if your mom (or another close blood relative) had it, you are at least somewhat more likely to have angle closure as well.

Angle closure glaucoma is more a disease of higher than normal eye pressure than is open angle glaucoma. As discussed in a previous section, the process of angle closure means that the iris moves to block the trabecular meshwork, raising eye pressure and causing damage. This can happen either suddenly (an acute angle closure crisis) or more commonly as a silent but off-and-on process that gradually plugs up the meshwork with iris stuck to it, leading to a chronic disorder. The dominant reason for the iris to block the meshwork is that it starts out close to the outflow area in the first place in smaller eyes. Smaller eyes are often "far-sighted" (hyperopic). Persons with hyperopia develop the need for eyeglasses in midlife and become unable to read print without glasses earlier than everyone else. When we measure the length of their eyes, they are shorter than average, with crowding of the structures together. This slows the movement of aqueous humor from where it is produced behind the iris (at the ciliary body) through the pupil (between the iris and lens) and into the front chamber (anterior chamber) of the eye. Because the block of aqueous movement is at the pupil, doctors call it pupil block. If there were an opening in the iris, the fluid couldn't be blocked—so the first treatment for angle closure is to make a hole where there isn't one naturally. This is done in the office with a laser, pretty painlessly, with only eyedrop anesthesia (laser iridotomy, see **Laser glaucoma surgery: iris holes and angle treatment**).

More detail about the risk of developing angle closure glaucoma and treatment or no treatment for suspects for angle closure is included in the section **Why isn't glaucoma either there or not there—what makes you an angle closure suspect?**

I have never been told ... in 20 yrs ... whether I am "open" or closure!"

Will you go blind?

TAKE HOME POINTS:

- **Odds of going blind are low**
- **Once damage happens it can't be fixed**
- **Relatively more blindness from angle closure than open angle glaucoma**
- **We must prevent damage before it happens**
- **Adherence with the treatment program improves your chances**

If you are like many persons that we have cared for, one of the first thoughts you have when presented with the knowledge that you have glaucoma is: will I be blind? The good news is that if you are not blind at this time, there is a very good chance that you will never be blind, at least from glaucoma. It is true that glaucoma is the second leading cause of blindness in the world after cataract. And, it presents a real threat to the vision of anyone who develops it. But from scientific studies all over the world and among persons just like you, we can say that the vast majority of persons who know that they have glaucoma, and who continue to follow the standard care instructions, will arrive at the end of their lives still reading and seeing well enough to enjoy life from both eyes.

Once we are adults, we don't grow any new cells in our brain. Since glaucoma kills nerve cells that are truly part of the brain, it is not surprising that once vision is lost from glaucoma, it cannot be restored. The nerve cells that are dead were part of an intricate network in the retina and had a long fiber stretching inches up into the brain to begin a visual process that is more complex than we can even imagine now. Our best hope for the glaucoma patient, and the goal of treatment, is to save the vision that is left. We can do that to such an extent that most of those with glaucoma will live normal visual lives. Research in our laboratories and in others is presently working very hard to find ways to restore lost vision from glaucoma and other diseases (see the next section **Can glaucoma be cured?**), but at present nothing can be done to return vision that has been lost from glaucoma.

Actual statistics show that about 5% of European-derived persons with glaucoma will lose the ability to read standard print in both eyes from open angle glaucoma. The number is 3 times higher among African-Americans. And, it is also 2-3 times higher for those with angle closure glaucoma. But, many of this small percentage who become blind are those who were nearly blind before they found out that they had glaucoma. A famous glaucoma specialist from Boston, Morton Grant, wrote about his many years of seeing and studying glaucoma. He concluded that those few patients who did badly and lost their vision from glaucoma were most often those who didn't follow care instructions or who came to the doctor too late. For the persons in that group, we have included a section **What does low vision treatment have to offer?**

Again, looking at real statistics, about 15% of glaucoma patients will lose the ability to read in one eye. That is a tragedy for them and hurts their ability to do some things that require vision to see in 3 dimensions, what is called depth perception. Having lost one eye, one is more likely to knock over the salt shaker at dinner, or to stumble on stairs and curbs. Glaucoma damage decreases the contrast sensitivity of the vision system, so what seemed like a black and white page of print before is now more grey and white. Glare is more of a problem for the glaucoma patient. And, you must develop methods to adjust to changes in lighting when moving from bright sunshine to dark interiors, or the other way around. Each of these effects is due to the loss of some ganglion cells from the retina in the eye.

Glaucoma is most likely to affect one eye much more than the other. We don't know why this is, since both eyes have seemingly been exposed to the same environment, diet and use. My mom went to the orthopedic surgeon with pain in her right knee. She asked the doctor: "why is my knee hurting?" and he answered: "Well, Mrs. Quigley you're 80 years old." She said: "The other knee's 80, too, and it doesn't hurt!" But, it turns out to be fortunate that glaucoma affects one eye more, since damage mostly in one eye with the other eye unaffected leaves the person pretty functionally normal. Our research at the Glaucoma Center of Excellence has been instrumental in showing how glaucoma affects persons' lives in the real world. Those with one eye that is largely intact can do most daily activities as well as persons with two good eyes. While they must maintain a higher level of alertness, driving and walking are largely done just as well and safely by early and moderate glaucoma patients as their equal aged brothers and sisters with two good eyes.

The areas of vision affected by glaucoma are fortunately not in the center part of our world where we read and watch televisions and computers. The zones where the early dying nerve cells see the environment are in the middle areas, not the center and not at the extreme outside of our peripheral vision. Since the brain normally gets input from both eyes about every place in our immediate world, as long as one eye is providing the picture of a zone, the brain isn't missing anything. This explains something that puzzles patients when they see their visual field testing from each eye. The doctor shows them black areas (areas where the eye cannot see) in one eye, yet as far as the patient is concerned there are no such black areas or missing spots in their real world when they are looking with both eyes. That's good for continuing to function normally, but it is one reason why people don't notice their own glaucoma damage until very late in the injury process. If the left eye still sees what the right eye is missing, damage in the right eye is not noticed. And, the damage happens so slowly that the person has time to adjust to the change without realizing it is happening. When we measured those with severe glaucoma damage in both eyes on a walking course, the person bumped into things more and walked more slowly than those of the same age. When we asked them if they had any trouble walking, they said: "No"—because they had realized gradually that walking had become more difficult, but had taken it for granted that it was due to old age.

There is very active research to determine what effects glaucoma has on important activities of daily living. We often hear from patients that they are having more difficulty with reading, for example. When we measure their acuity on the letter chart on the wall, they have normal 20/20 vision. Perhaps the subtle loss of nerve cells near the central vision, or other effects of glaucoma, do actually impair reading. We have determined that glaucoma patients can start reading at a normal pace, but slow significantly within 15-20 minutes. Glaucoma patients also give up driving earlier than persons of the same age without vision problems. Driving a car is a vital personal activity that determines in many ways the ability to live independently in our society. We need to determine which patients should, in fact, stop driving, and which ones can continue to do so safely.

While it is true that most glaucoma patients don't get to a stage of severe vision loss, there is a slow worsening of vision function in some glaucoma patients with time, even when appropriate treatment is given. This worsening is so minor in the majority that we can feel confident they will not be impaired in their lifetime. But, a minority of those with glaucoma progressively worsens at a rate much greater than the rest. For the slow progressors, standard treatment is perfectly sufficient, while for the rarer ones with more aggressive disease, treatment must also be aggressive. As we deal with the examining techniques and treatments for glaucoma in the next sections, it will become clearer that "one size doesn't fit all" for glaucoma treatment. Some need only regular examinations and don't even need pressure lowering therapy, while others must undergo surgery to save vision. But, whichever group one falls into, vision should be able to be saved with a good program jointly agreed to by doctor and patient.

Can glaucoma be cured?

TAKE HOME POINTS:

- **There is presently no cure**
- **Successful treatment can stop meaningful vision loss**
- **Nerve cell replacement research has taken initial steps**

When she was 90 years old, my wonderful Grandma Mamie told me she was having trouble putting on pullover sweaters because her shoulders had arthritis. "Harry," she asked, "you're at that medical school Johns Hopkins, when is my shoulder going to get better?" I had to help her understand that we weren't going to cure her shoulder, but we could buy her button-up sweaters. An important part of helping persons with glaucoma is to channel that hopefulness that Mamie expressed into flexibility to deal with what they've got. (Mamie kept winning at Bingo and playing bridge for some time afterward).

In this section, we'll discuss two forms of definitive treatment for glaucoma, one may happen in the future, and one is what we can do now. The future hope is to restore vision that has been lost. That can't presently be done. The present treatments can slow the process so much that no meaningful loss occurs in the person's life-time. Successful glaucoma surgery can lower eye pressure to a safe level (**Operations for glaucoma**). Such surgery can last for many years without need for any eye drops or medicines. But, since there are some surgery eyes that start needing medicine or more surgery again later, it is important to keep having doctor's exams regularly even when successful surgery has been done. So, checkups will be needed, just as they are for other serious illnesses where a remission has been produced, to be sure it doesn't come back. For now, we have several ways to lower eye pressure to really slow vision loss from glaucoma.

As described already, the successful treatment for most persons with glaucoma is to take daily eye drops indefinitely. Several laboratories and companies are presently working on a variety of ways that the medicine for glaucoma could be given only once or twice per year. These approaches will probably include placing the medicine as a deposit under the surface of the eye or even inside the eye in the doctor's office under sterile conditions. This may sound scary, but for another eye disease called age-related macular degeneration, inside the eye injections every month are already proving to be a sight restoring method that older persons find easy to tolerate. This could really increase the number of those with glaucoma who no longer need to take eye drops every day.

There are several things that could be placed on or in the eye that could help. Some would be drugs in a long-lasting formula that lower eye pressure. Others would be carriers made from modified virus particles that get inside the eye cells in the front or back of the eye. Once inside these viral carriers fool the cells into thinking that the DNA they carry should be translated like a normal gene and the substance that is produced is made by the cell as if it were a natural molecule. The Glaucoma Center of Excellence team has already tested several such molecules that slow glaucoma damage in animal models of glaucoma. Ideally, one injection of such a viral carrier would last for years to protect the eye. This may sound like Star Wars, but one eye disease called Leber's congenital amaurosis has already been helped dramatically in human eyes by this type of approach. People with that disease have the fortunate situation that when the viral carrier was injected, they actually saw better. This insertion of

48

DNA is called gene therapy, and there are active research programs to use this approach for glaucoma.

Gene therapy is only one of the things now being included in the approach called neuroprotection research for glaucoma. This type of treatment, when it becomes available, will involve any method that keeps nerve cells alive longer—and preserves the vision that the person has at that time. But, gene therapy and neuroprotection will not restore lost vision. In general, these methods do not try to lower eye pressure, but rather they make the eye or the nerve cells less likely to suffer from the effects of eye pressure and the other negative things that glaucoma does. We now have more than a dozen types of potential neuroprotective drugs that have been shown to work in this way in mice, rats, and even monkeys. One full trial of a drug called Memantine in over 1,000 patients was conducted to see if the pill would slow the rate of peripheral visual loss in glaucoma patients. The drug didn't work well enough to be recommended for patients with glaucoma, but some large drug companies are actively researching this area. A very small study tested whether one of our existing eye drops for glaucoma has additional benefit as a neuro-protectant. Unfortunately, the data require confirmation before we can be sure what was found. When we talk to glaucoma patients and their families, there is often a wonderful hopefulness that adding some treatment to the standard approaches will be helpful. Consideration of the things that are called "alternative therapies" is given in section **Are there treatments other than lowering eye pressure?**

Standard glaucoma treatment has been shown to slow the progress of the disease in the majority of patients to such an extent that they never become more impaired than they are at the time they discover they have the disease. That isn't a cure, but it is a comfort. But, for those who have very significant vision loss from glaucoma, the hope is that we will find a way to restore vision. For some eye problems, there are actual improvements to be expected from treatment. Cataract means that the lens inside the eye has become clouded. Surgery is commonly done to remove the foggy lens and replace it with an artificial one. Cataract surgery routinely restores normal vision to those for whom cataract was their only problem. Yet, in glaucoma, the loss of vision is due to death of the nerve cells called ganglion cells. These cells do not replace themselves as our skin cells do, for example.

So, to be able to restore vision, we must put back a lot of nerve cells. And, they can't just be thrown into the retina, they have to go in the places where previous ones lived. And, they have to link up on one end with the other retinal nerve cells they normally get information from, as well as to grow a fiber along those 2 inches up to the brain, and link up with the partner cells in the next relay station. And, the connections (synapses) need to be made in a way that produces useful vision images, without messing up the existing connections for the parts of vision that haven't been lost from glaucoma already.

As you can see, that's a lot of "And"s. But, 10 years ago, I held a meeting of scientists in which all the group talked about was how impossible it would ever be to restore vision in glaucoma. My lab and other research groups went to work and since then we've accomplished some of the initial steps. First, we know where we can get the nerve cells that we need—we can get them from your own eye. Within every eye are cells that made lots of daughter cells during life in the womb, then when the eye was "finished", they went to sleep and stopped dividing. They're alive, in the front part of the eye (the ciliary body), where we can get some out (surgically) without hurting the eye (Figure 9). Thousands of new cells can be made from such a piece of removed tissue, and the beauty is that they are your cells, so there shouldn't be a problem with rejection. That's when someone else's tissue is put into you and is attacked and killed since it's foreign.

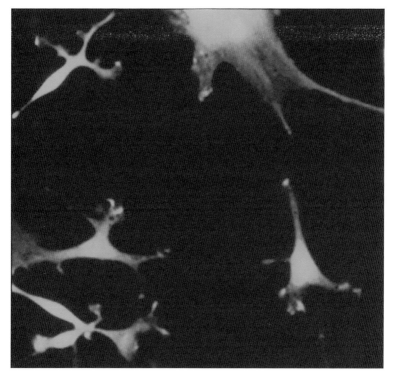

Figure 9: New progenitor cells that were produced from existing cells in an eye, shown growing in a culture dish. These may someday become the replacement cells that could restore vision lost from glaucoma.

These new cells from inside the eye are called progenitor cells. They went pretty far toward becoming eye cells during development prior to birth, then they stopped developing and stayed quietly in the eye, waiting to be turned back on. Why don't we want to use stem cells, which you have probably read about? Scientists call something a stem cell when it can turn into many different things, like a bone cell, an ear cell, or a heart muscle cell. Stem cells are present in fetuses at an early stage after fertilization and we have learned a lot about development from them. But, there are ethical and practical issues involved in their use when they come from unborn fetuses. Other "stem cells" have been produced by treating adult cells in special ways. For these and for fetal stem cells, we would have to convince the stem cell that it wants to be an eye cell.

51

Instead, the approach we have taken is to start with a progenitor cell that already had begun to be an eye cell. Furthermore, stem cells come from a different person and the body's attempts to reject them would need to be treated.

Progenitor cells from the eye and from some other tissues (like the bone marrow where blood cells start) have been tested as replacements in the eye and there are some positive results. Progenitor cells have been convinced to move into the retina of animal eyes and have lived there for brief periods. No one has yet succeeded in finding a way to take the next steps: getting the synapse connections wired up to the existing cells in the retina and growing a fiber up to the brain. We have plans that hopefully will beat those problems. But, more work is needed and no therapy will be available for a number of years.

What tests are needed to diagnose glaucoma?

TAKE HOME POINTS:

- **Measure eye pressure (tonometry)**
- **See if angle is open or closed (gonioscopy)**
- **Test side vision (visual field test or perimetry)**
- **Examine optic nerve head (ophthalmoscopy, photography, imaging devices)**

So, if persons with glaucoma rarely find it themselves by noticing something wrong with their eyes, how does an eye doctor find it? The answer is through careful examining and good detective work. First, we look for those contributing risk factors that make it more likely that you might have either open angle or angle closure glaucoma. If you have two or three of these risk factors (such as having a blood relative with it, or being an older African-American who is near-sighted), it's mandatory to do the detailed exams for glaucoma that we'll discuss here. Why not just do all the tests on everyone? In every eye exam, the doctor asks questions about risk factors (called taking a history). The doctor also measures your eye pressure and looks into the eye at the optic nerve. But, it is a waste of time and money to perform all the other tests on everyone, because many people are at very low risk of glaucoma.

Tonometry

Eye pressure measurement is most often done with a tool called a tonometer (Figure 10). The tonometer used most now was invented by Hans Goldmann, a Swiss eye doctor who invented many other important diagnosis tools for glaucoma. This instrument is part of the big machine that is attached to a chin rest device that slides up in front of the patient with a pair of binoculars for the doctor to see things magnified and with a bright light. After numbing the eye with eye drop anesthesia, the Goldmann tonometer presses against the eye. The force with which the eye pushes back is used to estimate the pressure inside the eye. The tonometer is highly accurate and is the "gold standard" for glaucoma. Patients should not hold their breath during measurement (you can slowly breathe through your nose). For most patients, the eyelids have to be held out of the way with the doctor's (or technician's) fingers or they will make the measurement impossible—or worse, they can artificially raise the measured pressure by pushing on the eye.

Readings were not consistent when taken by Tech & then by Doctor.

I insisted they only be taken by the Doctor

Generally, the Tech was higher and different Tech's used.

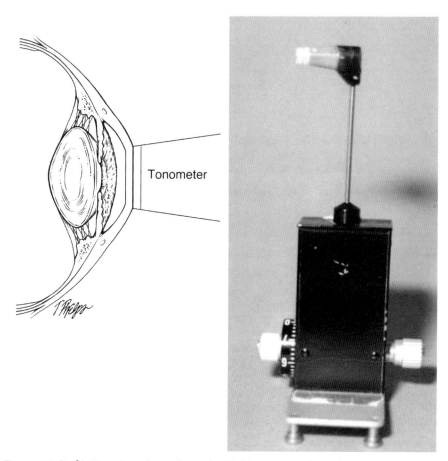

Figure 10: (Left): Drawing shows how the Goldmann applanation tonometer rests against and flattens the cornea to measure eye pressure. (Right) Photograph of the tonometer with its tip (top of instrument) that contacts the cornea.

Tonometry is usually easy to go through, since the eye has been numbed by drops, so you feel nothing. During the actual measurement, the instrument can rub some cells from the cornea if it is not done gently. If the patient rubs his or her eye during the 20 minutes afterward, the cornea can also be it scratched. This rarely happens, but can cause substantial pain or a feeling like something is in the eye. The doctor should be made aware if this happens.

Pressure was originally measured using the change in a column of mercury that we now only see in temperature thermometers.

WHAT TESTS ARE NEEDED TO DIAGNOSE GLAUCOMA?

Although the instruments have changed, the unit of measurement for pressure is still the same, and the range of normal eye pressure is from about 10 to 20 in units of millimeters of mercury. But, pressure measuring doesn't tell us who has glaucoma very often. Those who have open angle glaucoma only have a pressure outside the normal range half the time. The other half of those with pressures higher than normal doesn't have glaucoma (and may never develop it). So, having a higher than normal pressure is a contributing risk factor, and should lead to a full detailed glaucoma evaluation, but it isn't glaucoma. Those with angle closure glaucoma more often have higher than normal pressure, but not always.

Eye pressure varies a bit during an average day and from day to day. It can range 4 millimeters of mercury up and down in those with untreated glaucoma. It is, on average, higher first thing in the morning and lower in the evening, though this is not true of every person. It is higher when we are lying down than when we are standing (mostly this relates to how high our eye is compared to our heart). Hanging upside down or doing headstands, for example, causes eye pressure to go much higher (see section **How should you change your life?**). There is some evidence that greater variation in eye pressure may be worse for glaucoma patients. Some doctors advocate trying to estimate the degree of variability by measuring patients more often, on different days, at different times of day, or throughout one whole long day of measuring (called diurnal measurement).

Recently, newer tonometers were invented to solve problems that come up with pressure measuring. First, the Goldmann tonometer is hard to use when the cornea (the clear front of the eye) isn't normal in shape. Second, we've known for a long time that the pressure reads differently depending on how thick the cornea is, called central corneal thickness or CCT. This is measured with a small instrument called a pachymeter. The normal cornea is as thick as 5 pages of a book stacked together (about half a millimeter), and the tonometer depends on the cornea being that thick to be accurate. If your cornea is half a page thicker or thinner than the average, eye pressure will read differently. Thinner corneas read too low and thicker

① usually during same period ... of "factor applied".

② Not aware of ever being measured.

ones read too high. Persons with thinner corneas have been shown to be more likely to develop open angle glaucoma when they start out as suspects (see section **How did you get glaucoma?**) While several new instruments have been designed, they all have issues that keep them from being perfect enough to avoid these problems. The new instruments have disadvantages of their own (like being much more expensive to use). Of course, the doctor and patient want to have the best reading on what eye pressure is, so accurate tonometry is important. But, it is even more important to know how much the pressure has been changed from before therapy to afterward (see section **What is the target pressure?**). That is much less dependent on having the exact true eye pressure and more dependent on having lots of pressure measurements.

One new tonometer, the ICare has solved some problems well. It can measure pressure without putting in anesthetic drops, so for patients who are allergic to those drops we can now get a good reading. Equally important, we can get good pressures in infants and children much more often with this tonometer. That means fewer times when a child must be put under anesthesia to find out what their pressure is (see section **Children and glaucoma**)

TAKE HOME POINTS ON TONOMETRY

- **Applanation measurement is the present gold standard**
- **Having "normal" pressure doesn't mean you don't have glaucoma**
- **Having higher pressure doesn't mean you do have glaucoma**
- **Eye pressure varies through the day and night, more in those with glaucoma**
- **Thickness of the cornea affects pressure measurement**
- **There is a new tonometer that doesn't need eye drop anesthesia**

Gonioscopy

The second test done for all glaucoma patients is to look at the angle, where aqueous humor leaves the eye (Figure 11). Because the angle is inside the eye, essentially around a corner on the interior, it needs to be seen with a big contact lens called a gonioscope. There are several types of gonioscopes, but all are placed against the eye after it is numbed and have mirrors to allow the doctor to see several things. First, is the angle open, closed or somewhere in between? The angle runs all around the eye in a circle, so all 4 zones (up, down, nose side, temple side) must be looked at by turning the gonioscope (or having one with 4 mirrors). Second, doctors look for places where the iris has permanently stuck to the meshwork. These are signs of past, significant angle closure. Third, we look for other signs of abnormality, like new blood vessels or torn places from past injury, causing **Secondary glaucoma**.

I do not even remember having !

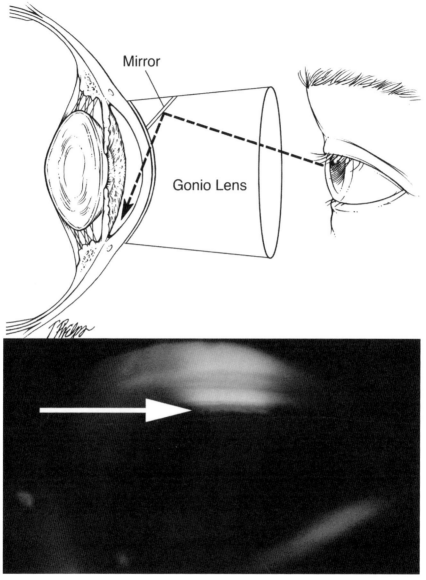

Figure 11: (Top) Drawing of how the doctor views the angle by bouncing light from a mirror in the gonioscope into and back from the angle. (Bottom) Photograph of an open angle as it is seen by gonioscopy (arrow shows the angle).

Unfortunately, eye doctors don't always do gonioscopy when it is appropriate, as our researchers found when we studied the charts of glaucoma patients from across the United States. Almost half of these charts did not have any documentation that the doctor had done gonioscopy or knew if the angle was open or closed. Patients who are glaucoma suspects or who have glaucoma will want to ask their doctor what their gonioscopy shows.

Gonioscopy is the main test that tells whether angle closure is likely. It isn't an all or nothing decision, and no eye doctor can classify every angle for certain. In probably more than 95% of all eyes, we could get 3 eye doctors to agree about whether an angle is open or closed. But, it is in the few in-betweeners that we must use judgment and make a joint decision with the patient about the best course. The decision in the case of angle closure is whether to make a laser hole in the iris immediately or to wait and watch to see how the eye does without laser iridotomy. Detailed discussion of this issue is in the section **Why isn't glaucoma either there or not there—what makes you an angle closure suspect?**

For some years, glaucoma centers like the Wilmer Institute have added newer exam methods to evaluate the angle to their gonioscopy. The most recent and promising of these is called anterior segment optical coherence tomography, or ASOCT (Figure 6). It is a painless imaging test that requires no anesthesia and has a dim light that reflects from the eye and makes a picture of the cross-section of the angle along with the cornea and iris. Our research with this technique has shown that the iris acts differently in those with angle closure—it is less "spongy" is one way to describe it. We and others are now looking for ways to show scientifically that using the new imaging methods will tell us much more about who needs a laser iris hole and who does not.

I have never seen an Image like fig 6.

> **TAKE HOME POINTS ON TONOMETRY**
>
> - **The doctor should evaluate the angle in every possible glaucoma patient**
> - **Most often the angle is open**
> - **Angles that are narrow or closed may need to have a laser iris hole made**
> - **Gonioscopy is not always certain to give the answer and newer methods are in development**

Ophthalmoscopy

The third important exam method used to identify glaucoma is looking at the retina and optic nerve head for signs of glaucoma damage. In this exam, called ophthalmoscopy, doctors look for signs that structural loss of ganglion cells and their fibers has already happened. Ganglion cells are scattered all over the retina, and their fibers converge on the optic nerve head like roads coming into a big city. The layer of fibers gets quite thick just at the nerve head and as the fibers pile up and dive into the opening. The nerve head, often called the disc is mostly filled with fibers. There is left over space in the middle of the nerve head called the cup, and the fibers are grouped around the cup in the rim. We all want to have lots of fibers, so we want a big rim (and by subtraction, a small cup). When we compare the size of the cup to the size of the whole disc, we talk about a "cup to disc ratio" (Figure 12). The bigger the ratio, the more empty space there is in the nerve head. That space may be left behind when nerve cells die. Most persons in the population average a cup/disc ratio of about 0.4, and ratios of 0.7 or greater happen only 2.5% of the time, so the ones that are this big raise suspicion that glaucoma might already have started (Figure 12).

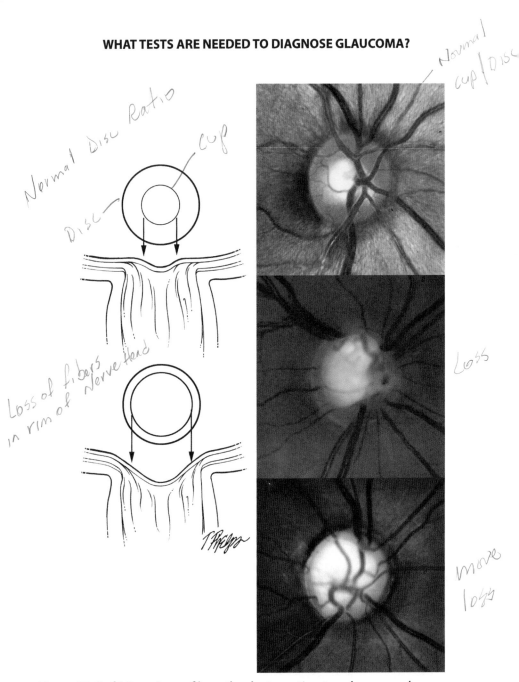

Figure 12: (Left) Drawings of how the doctor estimates glaucoma damage from optic nerve head examination. The outer margin of the disc determines the outer circle and the cup size determines the inner circle. The ratio of cup size to nerve head size is the cup/disc ratio. The upper left drawing shows a smaller, more normal cup/disc ratio and the bottom left shows a larger

cup/disc ratio due to loss of fibers in the rim of the nerve head. Top right: Photograph of a normal nerve head, with small cup to disc ratio; Middle right: nerve head with larger than normal cup and loss of upper rim of disc; Bottom right: large cup/disc ratio due to substantial glaucoma damage.

Patients who are having ophthalmoscopy usually have the pupil dilated with drops for the exam to allow a better view and to let the doctor get a stereoscopic (two-eyed) image to see the optic nerve head in 3 dimensions. In some patients, it is possible to see the optic nerve head well without dilation. When it is necessary to use drops to dilate the pupil for this exam, the person may be more sensitive to light for a couple of hours and for those who still can read without reading glasses, their near vision is poor due to the drops for a while as well. The examining light is very bright, and while it is not danger-ous, the person often can't see well for a few minutes after the exam. This is like staring at a car headlight and looking away; right after-ward one sees only blobs of color that block our vision.

Glaucoma causes loss of fibers in groups that run together, so in looking at the nerve head, there is sometimes a tell-tale notch or local loss of fibers in one area of the rim, typically at the top or bottom (see Figure 12 and 13, notch at upper rim). Big differences between the two eyes in the size of the cup are also a way to identify glaucoma that has started in the eye with the bigger cup. And, occa-sionally, bleeding in little splinter-like streaks happens on the nerve head to indicate that glaucoma is active.

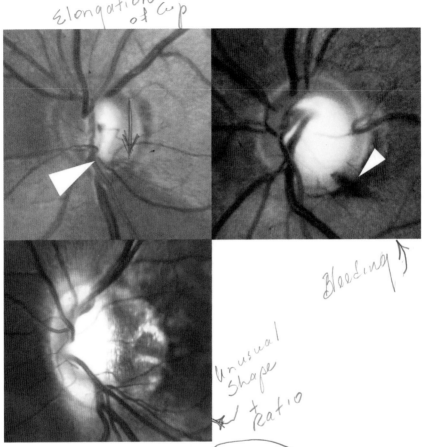

Elongation of cup

Bleeding

Unusual Shape

ratio

Figure 13: Photographs of nerve heads with glaucoma. Top left: cup extends abnormally to inferior rim of nerve head (arrowhead); Top right: bleeding on the inferior disc rim, seen as a flame-shaped red area (arrowhead); Bottom left: disc with unusual shape and larger than normal cup/disc ratio.

If the changes in the nerve head by ophthalmoscopy identify glaucoma, then why are some cases not diagnosed early enough? Perhaps the biggest problem is that the structure of the nerve head varies a lot among people. Many human features have a wide normal range. There are short people, 5 feet tall, and 7 footers, so just being outside the "normal" range doesn't mean that a disease is present. The cup can be big in some discs just because the disc itself is big and there's lots of left over space after the fibers go through. That leads to over-diagnosis of glaucoma in persons with big discs.

Small discs that start with no cup space can have real damage when the cup/disc ratio is in the middle of the average normal range. And, some discs have a tilted or distorted shape (Figure 13, bottom left) that makes judging the cup/disc ratio very hard, even though the eye sees just fine.

To add information during ophthalmoscopy, eye doctors started looked just outside the nerve head at the layer of nerve fibers as they came toward the disc to see if they were missing. This helps quite a lot with the unusual shaped discs to tell if there is fiber loss. But, this nerve fiber layer exam itself has variations and is harder in persons with light pigmentation than in darker individuals. The Wilmer Glaucoma Center of Excellence did a landmark study that showed one could predict functional glaucoma damage 5 years earlier by doing this nerve fiber layer exam.

For many years, it was most common to record how the nerve head looked by taking color photographs (as in Figures 12 and 13), often doing pairs of them to allow a stereoscopic view. These were repeated at intervals and the appearance of the nerve head as the doctor looked at it in the office was compared to previously taken photographs to see if the eyes were the same or had gotten worse. Color film gave way to digital photographs during the last decade in these cameras. But, these photographs needed to be taken with very bright flashes of light and with dilated pupils. The patient's vision is quite dimmed for a few minutes after this procedure and it is hard to drive home or see to read for some time afterward. There is still some role for this type of photography.

Both the need to have quantifiable information and the lack of convenience of color photographs has stimulated the development of digital imaging methods to assess glaucoma progress and stability. We now can measure the thickness of the nerve fibers with several such instruments, more comfortably and with greater ability to measure for change. Some of these instruments concentrate on the topography of the nerve head—kind of like measuring the slope in and out of a volcano's cone (Figure 14). Other instruments are good at estimating the number of nerve fibers and ganglion cells by making an optical thickness measurement (Figure 14). The true strength of these instruments has not been fully achieved yet, as their sensitivity is still being improved. The maximum help they give will be realized when we can depend on them to tell us if an eye's fibers have decreased quantitatively. That is an important measure of whether the patient is doing well (staying the same) or getting worse (losing fibers). There is considerable research being done to see which instruments allow us to judge how patients are doing.

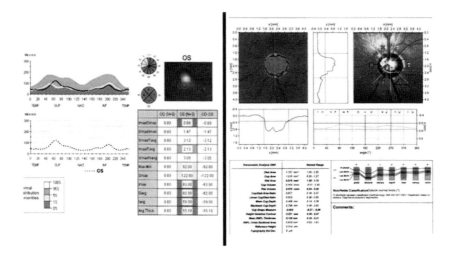

Figure 14: Images of the test result from digital imaging instruments for ophthalmoscopy. Left image is output from an instrument estimating the thickness of nerve fibers of ganglion cells around the nerve head. Right image shows printout from an instrument estimating the cup to disc topography;

TAKE HOME POINTS FOR OPHTHALMOSCOPY

- **Doctors look at the optic nerve head to judge whether loss of fibers has happened**
- **Glaucoma causes differences between right/left nerves, local fiber loss and tiny blood spots**
- **Variation among persons in nerve head appearance must be taken into account**
- **Nerve fiber layer loss seen both by the doctor and with instruments can improve diagnosis**
- **Change in optic nerve head appearance over time can be important**

Visual field test

The fourth test to diagnose glaucoma is the visual field test (also called perimetry). This test tells us if some vision has been lost. The test is done with an instrument that examines how each eye can see, looking one eye at a time. We cover the eye not being tested with a patch, and we must put an exact lens correction in front of the tested eye to get the best results. The patient looks into a dimly lit bowl-shaped area (Figure 15) and small oval lights appear briefly in different places in the field of view. The hardest part for patients is to keep looking in the center of the bowl while responding when lights appear in the side vision. The instrument records which lights you saw and didn't see by when you press a button. Our natural instinct is to look over at where the target light appears. But, that would show what you see directly in front, where our best, center vision is (the fovea). Since glaucoma affects the mid-peripheral vision early on, we need patients always to look at the center target during the test, so that we learn what damage may have happened in the area away from the center.

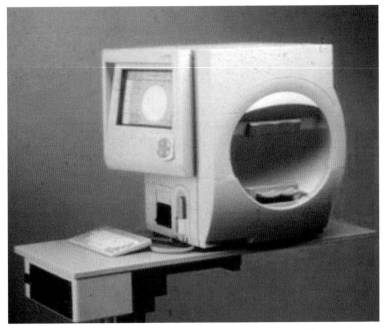

Figure 15: Photograph of one type of visual field testing machine.

The second difficult part of field tests is how dim many of the lights are. We want to see how dim a light the person can see, so we must show really tough to see ones. Furthermore, we have to test 55 or so locations to map how well you see in this area. So it isn't just whether you saw any old light, but how well you did at the extreme limit of your ability. I often say this is like weight lifting. You can probably lift 5 pounds, but if I keep adding weight, at some point you won't be able to lift any more. In a field test, that's when things actually get started. The machine wants to know what you can just barely lift. So it gets to the point where you can't budge it, then it takes a few pounds off so you can do it, then adds it back again until you can't again. The process is called finding the threshold—where you can just barely see the light half of the time. Naturally, you're going to think the test was hard. Just like the weight lifting test where I made you play around at your limit. In fact, during a field test the machine is trying to show you lights about 1/3 of the time that it knows you can't see. So you come away from the test thinking you've "failed".

68

People often say to me that they're sure that they have bad glaucoma damage after a field test. When I look at their test, it is totally normal for their age—they think they failed because they couldn't see every light, but that's exactly how the test is supposed to work.

Talk to your doctor about the field testing and especially ask how well you did compared to others your age (that's how it's scaled or judged, like "on a curve"). The first thing the doctor wants to know is whether your test in each eye is normal or not. After the first test, each test is then compared to the prior ones to see if there is any worsening. Unfortunately, it doesn't get better (at least not from present glaucoma treatment), although some people improve a bit just by having the test a second or third time—called the learning effect. Overall, our hope is that each patient stays as good as they were at the beginning of treatment.

Third, we learned 20 years ago that field tests that take too long to do are simply giving poor information about the patient's glaucoma. So, we have tried to speed up the test, getting it down to about 5 minutes per eye. There are even faster versions of the test for those with attention problems. Blinking normally is OK during a field test. If you find you need a rest, simply hold down on the response button to stop the test or ask the technician to pause the test.

To help us evaluate how you did on a field test, several "check trials" are done. One of these judges whether you were keeping the eye steady on the center target during the test. The technician can also see your eye on a T.V. monitor and may encourage you to look only straight ahead. Another check looks at whether you are responding when the target light isn't being shown. Everyone wants to do well on the test, since that would indicate the least amount of glaucoma damage. Our desire to "win" sometimes makes us over-respond. Again, the technical staff or doctor will point this out during or after the test and ask you to be "surer" that the light appeared next time. There are other more sophisticated checks done as well.

The vast majority of persons can give good information on field tests. But, the first test or two often are not so good—it takes practice to know what to expect and to give reliable answers. So, doctors must do 2 or 3 field tests to get a real baseline idea of where you stand. The technician in the room during the field test is critical to helping you get a good test. The room should be quiet (no cell phones ringing) and the technician should be attentive to how you're doing (and not going out for a break while you're sweating blood looking at lights). Sometimes the technician will gently move your head to keep it centered or pressed forward in the right position.

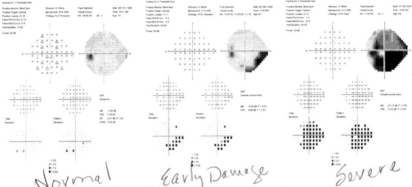

Figure 16: 3 printouts of visual field tests. The left test is normal, showing numbers for the sensitivity at various places in a circular test zone. Abnormal places are shaded darker. The bottom part of each printout compares your results to other persons of the same age. The middle printout shows early glaucoma damage, with abnormal, dark areas in the lower, right field area (black boxes). The right printout shows a severely affected glaucoma test—the majority of the picture is dark, meaning poor sensitivity.

By comparing your answers to those of hundreds of persons who did the test but were normal, the machine comes up with the likelihood that each point is either normal or not. So for each point across the whole field, we know how bad it is. Normal tests have no "black" areas, which are locations where vision isn't normal. Initial glaucoma damage is seen as a cluster of points just above or just below the horizontal horizon, most often on the side toward the nose (left of center in a right eye). As the disease gets worse, more areas turn black and the field of view can contract down so that only the very center of the world is relatively normal, along with a separate island of sight way out to the side of the temple (to the right in a right eye). Amazingly, even at such a severely damaged point, persons will sometimes not have noticed the damage and are surprised and unbelieving when we show it to them.

For some reason, one eye is usually hurt worse than the other in the field (about twice as badly). Of course this helps to maintain more normal function, since with one good eye we can do most activities of life without trouble. The average amount of worsening per year can be judged on the scale used for average damage, in units called decibels. The whole scale from normal to worst has 30 decibel units, and without treatment, the average person loses from 0.5 to 1 decibel unit per year after damage starts. With treatment, this is cut by more than half, so that over many years there can still be some loss, but not usually enough to be highly noticeable. The instruments now have software that shows graphs of how your fields are doing over time, and if things are getting worse faster than expected, this allows us to make a mutual decision to get more aggressive with therapy.

It would make sense that the fibers that are lost in the retina and optic nerve should have corresponding functional loss due to their absence. Because of the optics of the eye, the images on the retina are actually upside down compared to the real world, so when fibers that live in the upper retina and nerve head die, it causes loss of function in the lower part of the field test. In a perfect world, then, a glaucoma patient would have matching upper rim loss in the nerve head and lower field defects. When this happens, as it often does, the doctor can be confident that the finding is believable and should be taken as evidence for glaucoma damage. But, in a number of studies, persons who were moving from suspect glaucoma to established damage changed in their nerve head but not the field, or vice versa. Both examinations have variability that explains why this might be true. Therefore, doctors should be doing both kinds of testing, structural (evaluation of the optic nerve and nerve fibers) and functional (tests of the visual field), so that nothing is missed. In general, the structural change happens first, and the functional (field test) second. There are other tests that are sometimes used for glaucoma patients mentioned throughout this guide.

TAKE HOME POINTS FOR VISUAL FIELD TESTING

- It tests how well we see at the side of vision not in the direct center
- You're always going to think it's difficult and that you failed to see all the lights
- It often takes 2 or 3 tests to get good enough to give reliable answers (the machine knows)
- Early damage happens on the nose side of the field of view, above or below the horizon
- Progressive damage happens slowly enough it takes software to find it over several tests
- Matching the optic nerve head and field damage is a good confirmation method

Pachymetry: the measurement of central corneal thickness, using an ultrasonic probe held against the cornea with eye drop anesthesia. The importance of corneal thickness in measuring eye pressure and as a separate contributing factor to glaucoma is mentioned above in this section and in **How did you get glaucoma?**

Visual acuity measurement: letters read on a chart projected on the wall from big ones down to little ones, showing how good the center vision is. Sometimes a set of holes is placed in front of the eye to read the acuity chart. If the vision is better looking through one of the holes, this means that new eyeglasses would help the patient see better (called pinhole vision).

Ultrasonic biomicroscopy and anterior segment optical coherence tomography: instruments that show detail of the structures in the front of the eye and give information about movement of aqueous humor (see section **Why isn't glaucoma either there or not there—what makes you an angle closure suspect?**).

Afferent pupil response: The doctor shines a light on one eye then on the other. How the pupil responds as the light swings back and forth can tell that one eye's optic nerve is damaged more than the other.

How can you help your family avoid glaucoma damage?

TAKE HOME POINTS:

- Tell your family about your glaucoma and have them get good exams
- Specific gene mutations have been found explaining a few glaucoma cases
- There are no standard gene tests that help most patients now
- Present genetic research may provide new tests in the future

Several years ago, we did a study that asked 100 glaucoma patients to give us permission to call all their relatives and ask about glaucoma. We called 300 adult relatives of our patients and asked them what they knew about glaucoma, whether they knew they had a relative with it, if they knew it runs in families, and how often they had eye exams. Our results were disappointing. A lot of the family members did not know that they were at greater risk. The patients often hadn't told family members they have glaucoma. Some people aren't that close to family, and other patients said that they didn't think telling family members would lead them to do anything. "You know how grown kids are, they don't listen to me when I tell them to get eye exams", said one older patient.

Even worse, among the family members, more than half had never had a visual field test. Almost all of them said that they get their eyes "checked" every year, but they weren't getting the best test for finding glaucoma. We can't tell if that was because their eye doctor was choosing not to do the test or if he/she didn't know that the patient had a family history of glaucoma.

We tell every glaucoma patient to have all adult relatives (mother, father, sisters, brothers, adult children) go once a year to an eye doctor and say the following exact words: "My mom has open angle (or angle closure) glaucoma and I want a test of my angle and a visual field test." This makes sure that the correct tests are done and repeated every year. If you don't have glaucoma at age 40 or 50, it can still develop later, increasingly after age 60. It may be that glaucoma severity is also inherited, meaning that if you have a family member with severe vision loss from glaucoma, you are more likely to have that, too. People can't really be sure that their grandmother really had glaucoma without seeing the actual records from past doctors' exams. Having old records is very valuable.

It's one thing to say that a disease "runs in families" and quite another to know how the specific gene defects underlie the inherited tendency. Each gene functions like a recipe, telling the cell the ingredients needed to make a protein that your body needs. People have about 20,000 distinct genes, and scientists have only recently started to understand how some of them work. However, the process of looking for the "bad" genes has taught us some valuable lessons in medicine in the last 30 years. First, there is not one single gene that explains why people get a common disease. Glaucoma, like other complex disorders, has genetic factors, environmental factors, and other contributing features, so simple answers like a mistake, called a mutation, in one gene will not explain why most people get the disease. Second, when a defect in one gene is found in persons with a disease, there are often several areas of the same gene that can have mutations or changes that alter what the gene makes. If there is a mistake in the recipe, the protein can come out wrong, and there are many places where a mistake could be made. So, even within the same gene that is defective, it can malfunction in different ways in different people. Third, the disease-causing aspect can be how much product a gene makes rather than a defect in the gene code sequence for the molecule being made. Fourth, there are genetic disorders in which it takes two "hits" or gene defects in separate genes for the abnormality to happen (this is probably true for exfoliation syndrome (see **How did you get glaucoma ?**).

Hunting for genetic risk factors can be done by one of two approaches. Scientists look at the DNA of families with many members who have the disease, in a test called linkage analysis. They look for pieces of DNA that are linked to the presence of disease. In this method, the family relationships are very helpful for finding the gene, so the larger the family and more complete the information about who had the disease, the better. This method works best with rare mutations that greatly increase someone's chances of getting the disease. The other method, called an association study, doesn't use family information. In these studies, scientists compare the DNA of people who do or don't have the disease and again look for pieces of DNA more frequently associated with disease than you would expect by chance.

For open angle glaucoma, several likely zones in the human genome have been found, with 3 that have now been pretty well established to contribute to a small number of cases. Genes for the protein molecules called myocilin and optineurin are defective in certain subgroups of persons with open angle glaucoma. Myocilin mutations lead to high eye pressure at the age of 20 to 30 in families with this defect. Myocilin's action, when abnormal, seems to block up outflow of aqueous humor. Optineurin mutations are said to be more common in those with glaucoma at lower eye pressure. One hypothesis for how it causes damage is to make ganglion cells more sensitive to dying. For the subgroup with exfoliation syndrome, there are differences in a chemical coded by the LOXL1 gene, whose function relates to the supporting tissues in the eye.

One might think that genetic testing of blood samples might be a good thing to do, to determine if you have one of these defects. Practically speaking, however, the chance that the average glaucoma patient has one of the known mutations is really very low. The tests are very expensive (thousands of dollars per gene tested) and are not done in routine labs. Having the specific mutation or the variation in a particular zone (called a single nucleotide polymorphism or SNP) doesn't mean that you have a 100% chance of glaucoma. So, at this time, it is only in research studies that gene testing has value.

Why isn't glaucoma either there or not there—what makes you an open angle suspect?

TAKE HOME POINTS:

- **Formal definitions of two major glaucoma types have been suggested**
- **Definite optic nerve damage and functional loss = glaucoma**
- **Open angle suspects include those with higher than normal eye pressure, family history of glaucoma, or optic nerve heads that look like glaucoma**
- **People with high eye pressure (ocular hypertensives) get glaucoma only slowly**
- **The choice for or against treatment depends on gauging the risk and personal choice**

"So, Dr Quigley, if you've been studying and treating glaucoma for 40 years, how come you can't tell me if I really have it or not?" While not every suspect for glaucoma who I meet asks this question straight out, I'm sure it must occur to a lot of them, and it has been asked quite a few times. The truth is that very few diseases are 100% clearly there or not there. For example, an example of something that ought to be pretty straightforward is whether someone is alive or dead. I learned as an Intern that it's not so easy to tell. In the middle of the night, on a cancer ward, I was called from sleep by the floor nurse who said I should go into Mrs. M's room and "pronounce her" deceased. This nice lady had widespread cancer and I'd helped her through her last days. In the room, sitting at the bedside, I realized I hadn't been taught the "rules" of how to be sure someone was gone. I watched for breathing for a minute. I used the blood pressure cuff and stethoscope but heard no sounds of blood moving. So, I was pretty sure. But, when I listened for her heart sounds, I could still hear her tummy grumbling. It was nearly a half hour before I felt confident enough to sign the paperwork.

Diseases benefit from having very formal definitions. You may be aware that for life and death they sometimes use a test of brain electrical activity. But, until recently, both open angle and angle closure glaucoma had no agreed upon definitions of when they were present. This led to some doctors telling patients that they have glaucoma and others saying that they didn't, even though both doctors agreed on exactly what the structure and function of the patient's eyes were at the time. While there is room for judgment, a formal system was needed, and one was suggested by a panel that considered the issues and published their decisions in 2002.

The most important part of this glaucoma definition was to call it glaucoma only when there is measurable damage to ganglion cells, both structural and functional. This made formal a trend that most glaucoma specialists agree with now—namely, that we use the term glaucoma for damaged eyes, and call those in whom damage is either not present or might be present as "suspects". For open angle glaucoma, this means that the level of eye pressure is not part of the definition. Not that it isn't an important contributing feature, but we just don't call it open angle glaucoma because the pressure is "elevated" or "abnormal".

Open angle glaucoma suspects are suspicious for a variety of reasons. You may have a close blood relative with glaucoma. Your optic nerve head may naturally look similar to one affected by the early stages of glaucoma. In fact, there are a lot of people whose optic nerve head is big in diameter and these look to the eye doctor as if glaucoma has started, though it has not. Or, you may be one of the several million persons in the United States whose eye pressure is higher than the upper end of the average range (statisticians call this the 97.5 percentile, meaning only 100 minus 97.5 or 2.5% of people would have pressure that high). This is somewhere above 22 or 23 millimeters of mercury by tonometry, and puts someone in the category of suspects for open angle glaucoma that are called ocular hypertensives. For 10 years, our Wilmer Glaucoma Center of Excellence followed the health of nearly 1,000 ocular hypertensives. Some were treated with eye drops, and some were not treated. We found that the rate at which they developed definite structural and functional damage (i.e. they got glaucoma by the formal definition), was about 2 out of 100 persons for each year that we watched them. That surprised some people who thought that the risk would be much higher. In fact, when a formal study was done nationally (the Ocular Hypertensive Treatment Study), our finding was found to be accurate. Furthermore, in this clinical study half of the ocular hypertensive suspects were randomly assigned to take drops to lower pressure and half were assigned not to take drops. The rates of getting initial glaucoma per year were 2 in 100 in the untreated group and 1 in 100 in the treated group. We can conclude two main things: 1) treatment lowered the risk significantly, and 2) the risk is pretty low for the average ocular hypertensive suspect, treated or not.

Let's stretch out the time line for the ocular hypertensive suspect from when they first learn they have the problem (but not yet the disease) until when they are likely to die. Now I don't know when any one person is going to die, but insurance companies make a lot of money by knowing how likely you are to die. They use this date to price your premiums. The average person at age 65 who is generally healthy will live *on average* for 20 more years. So, at the untreated suspect rate of 2% per year, they have about a 20 times 2% or 40% chance of getting early glaucoma damage in one eye. The other eye will probably still be normal at that point. An 80 year old person will live less than 10 more years, so for them the risk of being untreated is a 20% chance of one-eye damage (10 times 2%). In general, when the doctor finds that initial damage has begun, the patient won't have been able to tell yet. None of us wants to lose any function at all, so some persons who are suspects tell me that they want treatment to cut down this risk, even though the risk is very small. Others (in fact the majority) say that the risk sounds pretty small, and we can just carefully monitor the eyes' status by ophthalmoscopy and imaging and visual field testing without treatment. This is particularly true for older patients.

Neither the suspect who chooses treatment nor the one who stays off treatment is making a bad choice. It depends on their actual risk (we'll get more detailed in a moment), and their individual risk tolerance. Patients often ask me: "Would you start treatment for ocular hypertension if it was you, Dr. Quigley?" Before I answer them, I ask them if they want to know what kind of risk taker I am. For example, would you jump off a 40 foot cliff into a river without knowing for sure how deep it is? I once (foolishly) did that as a young person. Perhaps that shows some part of my own risk tolerance. The point is that the best way I can give treatment advice is to provide the best information we have on your actual risk and then ask how you feel about those chances. It isn't the doctor's choice to make, though some doctors act as if they have the answer etched on a stone tablet. It's a shared decision.

I like to point out that people fall into different categories. Some people who are presented with the decision about treatment of their suspect status would go to bed every night convinced that they had lost another nerve fiber. They wouldn't enjoy life as much from the worry. For that personality type, trying treatment is a good option. Another group of persons seems less worried by the disease than by the side effects of treatment. They're convinced that drug companies are out to poison them (or at least to rob them) and they find the low level of worsening in untreated eyes to be not that scary. For them, careful follow up exams without treatment is the right choice. Yet, these two persons could have exactly the same statistical risk based on all the available information.

Asking which level of risk you can tolerate often helps to make the initial decision for a suspect patient. But, many others say: "I came to this big medical center to get your advice, so tell me what

your opinion is". If the decision is to be made mostly on risk calculation, then recent research based on the Ocular Hypertension study
and extended by our group at Wilmer is important to consider. As
we ticked of the contributing risk factors in the section **How did you
get glaucoma?**, several factors had a measurable impact on risk of
glaucoma damage. While the average untreated rate of conversion is
2%, there are those with less than 1% and some as high as 20% per
year. The factors that increase risk that we can use mathematically
to calculate the risk are: older age, higher eye pressure, larger cup to
disc ratio, worse visual field test outcome, and thinner central cornea. If we take the actual number values for these factors and plug
them into a formula for risk calculation, we can put each suspect on
a scale of likely worsening. Many doctors are now doing this routinely as they help patients with their decision.

There are other risk factors that aren't so easily incorporated into
formal risk calculation. This is because they weren't yet included in
the data collected in studies that measure their impact or because
they're hard to quantify. These include degree of near-sightedness
(myopia), presence of the exfoliation syndrome, having affected
family members, low blood pressure, and being of African-derived
ethnicity. Most eye doctors would increase risk for each of these
either a bit or a lot when someone has more than one.

Finally, we said that the risk is 2% per year, so if you are expected
to have 50 more years of life, your chance of having some damage
is expected to be 100%. This leads to the paradox that older age
increases the risk of developing glaucoma, but a 40 year old person
is more likely to develop damage than a 70 year old over the course
of their remaining lives—if both start at those respective ages with
the same level of other risk factors. So, we are much more likely to
recommend treatment as a good option for the young ocular hypertensive than the elderly one. It isn't that we don't love and care for
our senior citizens, especially now that I have signed up for Medicare
myself. But, a recent study showed that it simply isn't either cost
effective or good medicine to treat ocular hypertensives over age
65, given the small chance that they will ever have vision problems
that affect their lives. This illustrates the difference between a public

81

health view of treatment and a personal view. You may be a 75 year old suspect who has thought through all the issues and wants to take eye drop treatment despite hearing that it's not "cost-effective". On the other hand, if you're an 80 year old who's been taking drops for years and have very low risk, you may wish to discuss a temporary stopping of treatment with your doctor to see how it goes. Whether you choose treatment or no treatment, you're going to continue careful monitoring by ophthalmoscopy/imaging and visual field testing, regardless.

Monitoring.

I need to define "what is my state?

Which one Am I ?

Why isn't glaucoma either there or not there—what makes you an angle closure suspect?

TAKE HOME POINTS:

- In narrow angle suspects, the iris blocks the view of half or more of the meshwork
- Symptoms of past angle closure are an important sign
- With signs of disease (angle scars, higher pressure, acute crisis), it's angle closure, not suspect
- With damage to nerve head and field test, it's angle closure glaucoma
- Which angle closure suspects should get laser iris hole (iridotomy) is controversial
- All angle closure and angle closure glaucoma should have iridotomy
- Behavior of iris and choroid are probably contributing features in angle closure
- Plateau iris is a rare condition requiring additional treatment

In the section **How did you get glaucoma?**, we listed some contributing factors for angle closure and angle closure glaucoma. These included older age, being female, being of Asian derivation, and having smaller eye length. However, the key to the new definition system mentioned in the preceding chapter (sometimes called the Foster *et al* or ISGEO classification) is the appearance of your eye by the gonioscope exam (see **What tests are needed to diagnose glaucoma?**). Persons whose angles prevent a view of the trabecular meshwork through more than half of the angle in each eye are considered angle closure suspects. This means that the movement of aqueous from the back chamber of the eye to the front is blocked. Aqueous must come through the pupil opening and the lens is sitting right in the way in those who develop the actual disease. The way around the problem is to make a hole in the iris with a laser (Figure 17; for the actual technique description for the procedure, see **Laser glaucoma surgery: iris holes and angle treatment**). However, for every 10 persons with smaller eyes and narrow angles, only one will actually develop glaucoma. This means that small eyes and narrow angles are not the whole story and some other factors are contribute to the risk. Until recently, we didn't know what these additional features might be. Doctors were forced into a tough dilemma. They could treat everyone with narrow angles (and do 9 times too many laser iridotomies) or they could try to guess which one of the ten might get the disease, and potentially miss treating the right one—putting that person at risk for missing out on a preventive treatment that is largely curative at a pre-disease stage of the problem.

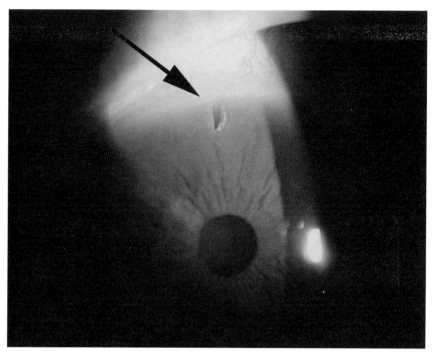

Figure 17: Photograph of an iris hole made with laser (iridotomy), a dark circular area on the upper part of the brown iris (arrow). The eyelid normally covers the treatment spot so that it is not visible to others, but here the eyelid was held out of the way.

Some eyes make the decision easier by showing that they don't just have a narrow angle, but bad things have already started to happen from it. These persons have a condition called angle closure. They've gone beyond being angle closure suspects. One of the signs that angle closure has started to affect the eye is the presence of areas where the iris has stuck to the meshwork in the angle and can't be pushed back during gonioscope exam (peripheral anterior synechiae). These happen by the following sequence (see Figure 7):

1) Narrow eye structures lead to a blockade of the aqueous moving between the iris and lens through the pupil

2) Pressure is higher behind the iris than in front of it, pushing the iris forward.

3) The iris bows forward like a sail on a sailboat to touch the meshwork

4) The iris stays against the meshwork so long that it is permanently scarred there.

The resistance to aqueous moving through from behind to in front of the iris is greatest when the pupil is neither big nor small—that is, when it is mid-dilated or about 5 millimeters in diameter. In the past, doctors tried to see if high eye pressure could be produced in suspect eyes by putting the patient in a dark room or dilating the pupil to 5 mm with drops—called provocative testing. Occasionally, these tests showed higher pressure, but recent research has pretty much shown that these tests don't simulate how angle closure happens often enough to be useful. The reason that many pills, both over the counter and prescription, are marked as dangerous for those with "glaucoma" is their ability to dilate the pupil and make angle closure more likely (see section **Can the treatments be worse than the disease?**).

When the movement of aqueous through the pupil is blocked off and on, the iris bows forward to stop fluid leaving the meshwork, raising the eye pressure intermittently. If this happens over and over, eventually the whole meshwork can be damaged, whether it is actually studded with scars of iris to meshwork or not. As a result, higher than normal pressure is another feature that moves the suspect to angle closure status. Notice that this is an exception to the rule for open angle glaucoma about eye pressure. In open angle glaucoma, the pressure can be high or low and the disease might still be present. In angle closure and angle closure glaucoma, the reason for the disease is (by definition) that the iris is blocking the meshwork and the pressure rises. So, most often we find that angle closure eyes have higher than normal eye pressure, and in the angle closure group, having a higher than normal eye pressure is a sign that the angle appearance is likely blocking the flow of fluid out of the eye.

Finally, if there is total closure of the angle, then the eye pressure goes very high and an emergency situation has happened. This is an acute crisis (also called an attack) of angle closure (see **Acute angle**

closure crisis). Some eyes have had smaller, past attacks and the eye got out of it by itself. But when this happens, there are tell-tale signs left behind for the doctor to see: areas of the iris get thinner and lose pigment, and the lens gets hazy areas. These are also reasons to consider that suspect status is over and real angle closure is present.

For all those with angle closure, especially those with the acute crisis, laser iridotomy should be done in both eyes. The evidence supporting this is very strong. Many years ago, when only the acute crisis eye was treated, attacks happened often in the other eye, and it was damaged needlessly. The approach of making a laser iridotomy in both eyes applies to all eyes with angle closure and to those angle closure patients who already have glaucoma damage (angle closure glaucoma). In angle closure glaucoma, it is very likely that further treatment will be needed with eye drops or even surgery after the laser iridotomy. People with angle closure and angle closure glaucoma should read the sections on eye drops and surgery, since they will probably be considering these therapies, too.

Why doesn't iridotomy cure the angle closure? As mentioned, the patient is typically not aware that the iris has been banging into the meshwork for months or years, causing damage to aqueous outflow. Laser iris holes stop further meshwork damage, and they almost completely prevent subsequent acute crisis, but they can't reverse existing angle damage. The eye pressure is not only higher, but more unstable in persons with this kind of angle damage and the eye pressure will often need treatment to prevent further nerve head and visual field damage after iridotomy.

There is still controversy about which persons who are simply angle closure suspects should receive laser iris holes. The "treat everyone" approach suggests that making the laser hole completely stops most long-term problems from angle closure. Laser iridotomy is an outpatient, generally comfortable procedure to go through. It has few side effects or long term bad consequences. The patient no longer has to worry that they will suddenly develop an acute crisis while on a cruise or trekking in Nepal. The alternative is the "treat very few" approach. Those who follow this philosophy argue that treating every angle closure suspect means 9 out of 10 treated persons are having laser treatment that is not needed—they may never develop the disease. Laser iridotomy is suspected to speed the development of cataract. Some persons after iridotomy suffer a bothersome glare sensation due to light passing through the laser hole, but this is uncommon. Once again, person who is an angle closure suspect needs to be included in the decision. Some persons would worry every day that they were going to have an attack. I have met patients who carried around in their purse bottles of medicine to treat an acute attack in case it happened. For these persons, laser iridotomy is a good choice, especially if they have multiple risk factors (a family member with definite angle closure, a person with intermittent eye pains, or those with two risk factors, such as an Asian female with small eyes).

For persons who are more bothered by the thought of having a needless laser surgery on the eyes, we hold off doing the iridotomy immediately and examine them twice a year for 2-3 years. Each exam includes gonioscopy to see if new scars have appeared in the angle, along with eye pressure measurement, as well as annual ophthalmoscopy and visual field tests. I have followed many persons in this way for the rest of their lives, without their developing any problem. If I didn't treat any angle closure suspects, I would guess right 9 times out of 10. Occasionally, one of the suspects who is being followed without treatment shows signs that angle closure has started (higher eye pressure, new angle scar), and then laser iridotomy is clearly appropriate. Rarely an untreated person could develop an acute angle closure crisis. The risk of this is certainly very low.

Research is actively being pursued at the Glaucoma Center of Excellence to determine better which of the angle closure suspects will develop a disease and need iridotomy early on. Part of our approach is to stop just measuring how small and how narrow the eye's structures are, and to challenge the eye by seeing how it performs when conditions are changed. We have moved from measuring anatomy to measuring physiology, looking at dynamic behavior. An important part of being able to do this is the development of new imaging instruments to look at the front of the eye. For 20 years, the test called ultrasonic biomicroscopy (UBM) added much new information about angle closure. But, it was limited in its view of the eye and not too convenient for looking at dynamically changing aspects of the iris and angle.

We worked with a company to test the anterior segment optical coherence tomography instrument (ASOCT). This allowed us to see how the structures inside the eye changed from moment to moment in eyes in their normal state, in an exam that is totally comfortable for the patient. Our dynamic approach is better than anatomic static measurement because it is like testing how fast a baseball pitcher can throw instead of measuring how big his arm muscle is. Dynamic measurements of the iris showed an amazing fact that had never been known in all the centuries that we've gazed at each other's eyes. As light falls on the eye, the iris muscles constrict to make the pupil small (otherwise, we'd be blinded by the light). In the dark, we want a big pupil to let more light in (to see those navy blue trousers in a dark closet). The new ASOCT machine can measure the thickness and area of the iris in the doctor's office with no anesthesia. It soon showed that the iris is like a sponge: it sucks up water in the eye when the pupil is small and squishes the water back out when the pupil dilates. If it didn't, the iris would be so fat that it might block up outflow of water in many eyes. When we measured the gain and loss of water from the iris in angle closure eyes, they failed to lose water when the pupil was big. Given that they have narrow channels for water to get out in the first place, this doubles their problem and is a contributing risk factor. A French research team has confirmed that angle closure patients who had an acute angle closure crisis were much more likely to have this feature of poor iris sponginess. Tests of iris volume loss are now being used in a number of advanced Centers to tell which persons should have an iridotomy and which should not. These tests will take several years of following persons before they have definitive results, but even now the data help us to inform patients better.

Just as the normal iris acts like a sponge and can have poor sponginess that contributes to angle closure glaucoma, the layer of the eye called the choroid can be a contributor as well. The choroid is the middle of 3 layers in the eye wall, outside the retina and inside the sclera. It provides nutrition to the retina through its many blood vessels. It is typically only one-fourth of a millimeter thick. Optical coherence tomography technology allows us to measure the choroid's thickness in living eyes without any pain or discomfort to the patient. We found that the choroid's thickness changes from moment to moment. The key point is if the choroid gets thicker, bad things can happen to the eye, especially to eyes with potential angle closure. If a hole hasn't been made in the iris, thickening of the choroid can make angle closure more likely to happen. In some angle closure eyes, when the choroid thickens, it can produce a very difficult to treat glaucoma called malignant glaucoma. Or, when a surgeon is operating on an angle closure eye, choroidal expansion (thickening) can make the surgery much harder. There is now good evidence that many eyes with angle closure have choroidal expansion as part of the reason that they develop the disease.

A small number of eyes with angle closure have a condition known as plateau iris, in which the iris looks flat as it comes up to the angle by gonioscopy. After we do iridotomy, the majority of eyes with angle closure have a more open angle appearance afterward. About one-third, however, don't look more open. Despite this, nearly all these "still narrow looking" angles don't close, don't lead into long-term angle closure or angle closure glaucoma, and they never have acute angle closure crisis. In fact, we make it a point to try to provoke attacks after iridotomy by dilating the pupil in every eye after iridotomy to show as best we can that the eye is safe from further high pressure. Rarely, when we dilate the pupil after iridotomy, the very high eye pressure happens again. This is called plateau iris syndrome and out of thousands of patients I've seen over the years, I can count on one hand the number of them with this syndrome. Most eyes with the plateau configuration won't be at any risk for later acute crisis. But, when this unusual plateau syndrome does occur, we change the position of the outer iris by a different laser treatment called iridoplasty. These plateau syndrome patients are also sometimes treated with eyedrops to keep the pupil small most of the time (pilocarpine), and occasionally, cataract removal surgery or glaucoma surgery is needed (trabeculectomy).

Acute angle closure crisis

TAKE HOME POINTS:

- **Acute crisis is a true emergency and needs attention immediately**
- **You or your doctor may have caused the crisis by doing something to dilate the pupil**
- **Symptoms: eye pain (headache), bad vision in one eye, red eye, pupils different sizes, nausea**
- **Immediate treatment is to make a laser iris hole (iridotomy in both eyes)**
- **Some are cured forever, but others need continued treatment after laser iridotomy**
- **Two special conditions need particular therapy: plateau iris syndrome, malignant glaucoma**

Acute angle closure crisis deserves its own special mention, as it is one of the few true emergencies in the glaucoma world. Of all of the forms of glaucoma, angle closure has a much greater chance to cause permanent vision loss than open angle glaucoma, and the acute crisis (frequently called an acute attack) probably accounts for a lot of this damage. The mechanism by which it happens was described in the preceding section (**Why isn't glaucoma either there or not there—what makes you an angle closure suspect?**). It happens to those with angle closure under the situation where aqueous humor movement from behind to in front of the iris is so blocked that the pressure behind the iris pushes it against the mesh-work and stops all aqueous outflow (Figure 7). Eye pressure can rise to numbers like 70 millimeters of mercury (compared to the normal 15). This is so high that permanent damage to ganglion cells in the optic nerve happens in days to weeks rather than the much longer, slower process of typical glaucoma.

It is the sudden increase in pressure that causes the severe symptoms of the attack. A link between the stomach and the eye causes an attack to be not only the worst pain that people ever remember having, but also it causes nausea and vomiting. Sometimes the stomach problem is so prominent that people go to an emergency room and the staff pays attention to that, thinking it is appendicitis, before realizing that the eye is the cause. Acute attacks also get mis-diagnosed as migraine headaches.

The eye symptoms of acute crisis are pain, poor vision in the involved eye, redness of the white part, and a bigger and irregular pupil shape. More than 90% of acute crises are in one eye only, but for one in 10 persons it happens in both eyes. In order to see if an eye problem is in one eye or the other, one should cover with the hand on one side then the other. In the excitement of being in pain, we often forget to do such simple things.

The things that can set off the crisis are those that can cause the pupil to move to the danger position, half-way dilated. These include stress and excitement, spending time in a dark place (such as a dimly lit restaurant), and being exposed to medications that dilate the pupil a bit. This happens during general anesthesia for surgery, since a drug that dilates the pupil (atropine) is given by anesthesiologists. If you have bad eye pain after surgery under general anesthesia, have an exam by an eye doctor immediately. Acute attacks can also be caused by the many pills that are given that can dilate the pupil while helping you with things like incontinence, sinus troubles, and upper respiratory colds. The Food and Drug Administration doesn't distinguish the various kinds of glaucoma in its warnings on drugs about "glaucoma", so if you are an angle closure suspect who has not had iridotomy, call your eye doctor before taking any of these drugs. Most of the time, you'll hear that it's fine to take them. After you have iridotomy, you can take any of these drugs safely. The final types of drugs that can cause acute crisis are those used in the eye doctor's office to dilate the pupil for examination of the inside of the eye. We've seen this a number of times over the years, and patients who have had dilating drops and have pain the night of the exam and especially into the next morning should go right back immediately to be checked. There are a group of medicines that can cause a very unusual form of acute angle closure in people who otherwise weren't at risk for it (they don't have small eyes or other risk factors for angle closure). One such drug is topiramate, a headache pill which is also used in epilepsy. Another group of drugs that can do this are some antibiotics (see the section **Can the treatments be worse than the disease?**).

If you think you are having an acute angle closure crisis, go to the office of an ophthalmologist (a medical doctor who does surgery and laser surgery) or to an emergency room that you are sure has an ophthalmologist on call to come there and see you. Most metropolitan areas have an "eye trauma" center designated where immediate, appropriate care would be available. Don't drive yourself there, get a ride or take a cab.

The immediate treatment for acute crisis will most often fix it in the first hour. The pressure is lowered by either eyedrops or by letting a small amount of aqueous out of the eye. This sounds gruesome, but you won't feel it and it immediately relieves the pain. Sometimes, in order to begin the lowering of pressure, a laser is used to treat the outer part of the iris to move it away from the meshwork to let aqueous out faster (laser iridoplasty). The vast majority of crises are relieved as soon as a hole is placed in the iris with a laser (Figure 17). This instrument, called a neodymium-YAG laser, can be focused inside the eye to make the iris hole, without making any incision or hole in the eye wall (cornea). There is a slight feeling that something is happening, but typically only eye drop anesthesia is needed. Several deliveries of the laser may be needed to make a hole about 0.5 millimeters in diameter. That's all it takes to relieve most crises. Occasionally, a second type of laser is used in very thick irises (called a continuous wave laser or diode) to thin things down before penetrating with the neodymium-YAG. High quality centers have both available to use. The opening is usually small enough that others can't see it from normal social distances. Those who get within 6 inches of your face for long enough to find the iris hole are people who know you well enough that they're concentrating on other things. Sometimes a small hole is made initially and it is made bigger a month later.

The other eye should have a hole made, too, though most persons want to wait a day or so to try to get back vision in the first eye. Putting it off for a long time is a really bad idea.

If the crisis has been going on for longer than a day (and you may not have been aware of it during that time) or if there have been preceding little attacks in the past that led up to this one, the laser iridotomy alone is not going to cure everything. There can be scars in the angle that won't go away, leading eye pressure to stay high. There may already be damage to optic nerve structure and visual field function, so that vision is never fully normal again. Haziness in the lens of the eye (cataract) may be already present or develop quite quickly after iridotomy due to the prior high pressure.

Some have suggested that removing the lens (cataract surgery) would be a good treatment for acute crisis. Since the reason for the crisis is severe blockage of fluid movement between the iris and lens, that is a correct statement, but removing the lens and replacing it with an artificial intraocular lens by surgery in the middle of an acute crisis is very difficult. Only the most experienced cataract surgeons, working at a center with extensive equipment to operate on the retina and vitreous inside the eye should even attempt this. On occasion, the acute crisis is not broken by laser iris hole and by medication—this then calls for forms of glaucoma surgery (see section **Operations for glaucoma**).

An uncommon type of glaucoma happens in some eyes that seem to have a typical acute crisis, but do not respond to standard laser iridotomy, with pressure remaining high. The doctor will see some special clues that this condition, called malignant glaucoma has happened. Malignant glaucoma got its name because it was difficult to deal with; it has nothing to do with cancer. It even happens sometimes in persons who are not at risk for typical angle closure. The mechanism involves a collapse forward within the eye of the gel called the vitreous that fills the back two thirds of the eye cavity. The best explanation at present is that the process starts, like typical angle closure, with choroidal expansion, and in these folks the vitreous collapses forward due to pressure behind it. The treatments start with laser iridotomy, but then additional types of eye drops, oral and intravenous medication, and often surgery to make a channel through the vitreous gel are needed to cure the problem.

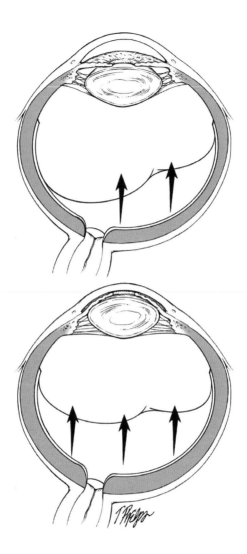

Figure 18: Drawings to illustrate the process that causes malignant glaucoma. starts with expansion of the choroid (shaded in grey, and thicker than the choroid in the normal eye (see Figure 1). The higher pressure causes aqueous to leave the front of the eye, causing a pressure that is higher in the back of the eye and lower in the front. Normal eyes can make the pressures equal by having water pass through the vitreous gel that fills the eye. Eyes with malignant glaucoma have poor water flow through the vitreous and it collapses forward, carrying the lens and iris with it until the angle is closed (lower drawing).

Low tension glaucoma doesn't exist and you don't have a brain tumor

TAKE HOME POINTS:

- **Open angle glaucoma often happens to those with normal eye pressure**
- **Low tension or normal tension glaucoma is not a separate disease**
- **Lower pressure glaucoma patients actually have a less aggressive disease**
- **It is not necessary (and bad medicine) to do brain imaging studies on those with typical glaucoma**

As described in previous sections, open angle glaucoma is no longer defined by the level of eye pressure. Studies of large populations in every continent on earth show that this disease affects many people with normal pressure as often as it does those with higher than normal pressure. In Japan, glaucoma at normal pressure is 80% of cases. But, until the 1970s, open angle glaucoma was known as the disease of "elevated" eye pressure and many experts thought that having it with "low tension" was a distinct disease. Not only was so-called low tension or normal tension glaucoma thought to be quite different, patients were often told that treatment by lowering pressure wouldn't work. Many patients still tell me that they have been told: "I've got that dread thing, normal tension glaucoma, and unfortunately none of the treatments will work. I'm going blind." But, we now know that among European-derived persons, 40-50% of those with open angle glaucoma always have normal pressure levels. It isn't that their pressure is irrelevant. Persons without glaucoma have eye pressures between 10 and 20—let's call this the "normal" range. When we study open angle glaucoma patients with pressures in this range, the eyes that are higher than 15 are more likely to be more damaged than those below 15. So, the higher the pressure in the normal range, the worse is the glaucoma. And, for those with glaucoma and pressure in the "normal" range, lowering the pressure with treatment is just as beneficial as lowering pressure in "high tension" glaucoma. There are only very modest differences between how glaucoma affects the optic nerve head structure and the visual field between those with lower and those with higher pressures.

Even more interesting, the most recent data show that those with open angle glaucoma at lower pressure (which I consider the right way to talk about this group) actually have a more slowly progressive disease on average than those with higher pressure open angle glaucoma. In other words, all other things equal, you'd rather have "low tension" than "high tension" glaucoma.

Among the most disturbing things that doctors used to do (and unfortunately sometimes still do) is to assume that a person with clearcut glaucoma-type damage to the nerve head and visual field loss might not have glaucoma because their pressure is normal. So, they order testing to find some other disease that might affect the optic nerve, like a brain tumor or multiple sclerosis affecting vision. On extremely rare occasions, a very atypical glaucoma-like set of findings turns out to be one of these disorders instead. But, good eye doctors know the features that define glaucoma, and those that define brain tumors affecting the optic nerve, and the differences are generally so clear that this additional testing is totally unnecessary. In fact, several studies have been done to show how silly it is to take people with typical glaucoma findings and subject them to the cost and inconvenience of brain imaging, lumbar punctures, and neurological consultations. The worst part of this is that it scares the patient in a way that they may never get over. If you were told that you "might" have a brain tumor or MS, hearing that they couldn't find anything on the imaging would never erase the "might" from your mind.

Over a decade ago, Dr. M. Roy Wilson, one of the most respected glaucoma doctors in the world wrote: "With respect to normal tension glaucoma, *there is no such disease* entity—distinct from primary open angle glaucoma—and it serves no useful purpose to continue to perpetuate this term." Yet, every year, doctors publish papers that are said to study "low tension" glaucoma. What could be done in such studies is to study everyone with open angle glaucoma and to treat the pressure level not as normal or abnormal, but as a continuous number from low to high.

What treatments are the right ones? Drops, scissors, laser

TAKE HOME POINTS:

- Any of the 3 pressure lowering methods works
- Side effects differ in each method
- Drops work for many, but produce side effects and require remembering to take them
- Laser has very low risk, but often isn't powerful enough in lowering pressure
- Surgery has reasonable success at lowering pressure, but a small number have bad effects
- Every method stops working in some eyes over time
- The method can be changed from one type to the other
- Decisions are shared by patient and doctor

In this section, we'll talk about the present mainline therapy for glaucoma, lowering the eye pressure. With due respect to the old game of rocks, scissors, paper, each has advantages over the other, but also each has a downside or two. The 3 methods are daily eye drops, laser treatment to the angle, or various forms of surgery. Which method to lower eye pressure is best for you to start with? This discussion applies whether you have open angle glaucoma, or you are an open angle suspect who chooses therapy, or if you have angle closure or angle closure glaucoma after iridotomy, and even for others with miscellaneous forms of glaucoma (see **Secondary glaucoma**).

The scientists in the crowd would say that all three treatments have been tested in big studies and they all work. Yes, that is correct. You wouldn't be wrong to start with drops, with laser or with surgery. The big organization that eye surgeons belong to, the American Academy of Ophthalmology, has guidelines called preferred practice patterns. These are written by committees that put together the best information for doctors to present to patients. The practice pattern says that every new glaucoma patient should be told the upsides and downsides of each of these methods, and that it's fine to start with any one of the three. Every new patient in our practice runs through the following discussion with us before the mutual decision about how to start treatment is made. So, what's the good news and the bad news?

Eyedrops: More patients begin treatment by taking daily eye drops than the other treatments. Perhaps this shows that patients think that medicines are safer than procedures. Perhaps it is because doctors have been most often telling patients that they should start with drops. It is true that many persons can have safe eye pressure lowering by taking daily drops. When we look at large studies, about half of those who start with drops will reach their goal pressure with taking one kind of drop per day, while another quarter will need two kinds of drops every day (two different bottles put in separately), and the final quarter will not find any combination of drops that works well enough and is tolerable enough for them to take.

The strong points of drops are that they usually don't do anything permanently bad to the patient or the eye, and they work as indicated the majority of the time. Also in their favor is that you can start them and if you don't like it, you can stop and switch to something else, mostly without any ill effects. The two weak points are: side effects and adherence problems. Soon after starting or in the longer term, some side effect or allergy can develop that keeps the drop from being usable. The specific problems with individual drop types are given below. Side effects vary from annoying and temporary to lasting and serious. Rarely, medicines for glaucoma can affect the heart and lungs and we know that a small number of people have even died from taking drops. But, it is surely true that more people have died from taking aspirin than glaucoma medicines. Our experience is that about 10% of people taking any eye drop will suffer a problem that forces them to stop taking it.

The second problem with taking drops is that we forget to take them or do not take them as prescribed. This is a much bigger issue than most patients believe. Once you know you have glaucoma, you will think that as a reasonable person, knowing your vision is on the line, you'll take the drops. You try your best. Unfortunately, careful observation of patients shows that it doesn't happen ideally. People who start the drops and fill some prescriptions will actually take drops on 3 out of 4 days. We'll deal with this issue in a whole section below (**How to succeed at eye drop treatment**).

Presently, there aren't ways to tell whether you will respond with a low enough pressure to a particular kind of drop. Some investigators have suggested extensive genetic testing to find out ahead of time who will have a good lowering from a certain type of drop. This approach is not presently possible and even though it sounds elegant, in a couple of weeks we can find out if your pressure fell by having you try a bottle, and that's cheaper.

Laser angle treatment (argon laser trabeculoplasty, ALT, selective laser trabeculoplasty, SLT, or laser trabeculoplasty, LTP): Almost 40 years ago, a brilliant doctor named David Worthen tried to lower eye pressure by shining laser energy at the meshwork in a controlled trial. Considering that he was working with advanced glaucoma eyes, the beneficial effect was pretty impressive, though small. Five years later, Dr. James Wise reported that when he treated fairly early glaucoma patients, their eye pressures fell impressively, and since then, a large controlled trial (the Glaucoma Laser Trial) showed that there is sustained lowering of pressure by this treatment as initial therapy. The meshwork runs all around the eye in a circle, so treatment generally is either half the circle or all the way around (360 degrees).

The good points of laser angle treatment are that it is nearly impossible to hurt vision or the eye when done properly, and, having laser treatment doesn't prevent a person from later using other treatments to lower eye pressure if the laser doesn't work. It's painless, takes only eyedrop anesthesia, takes about 15 minutes to do, and vision is nearly normal immediately.

However, a fair statement is that only half of those treated initially with laser will have sufficient pressure lowering that they don't have to do something else, too (such as taking daily eye drops). About another one-quarter get some lowering but have to start drops to get low enough. And, one-quarter get no good effect at all (though they aren't worse off either). Therefore, the biggest problem is that laser angle treatment isn't powerful enough. It works best for those with uncomplicated or primary glaucoma, and probably shouldn't be tried in those with secondary glaucoma (see **Secondary glaucoma**).

I am always amazed to hear from patients that they were told by an eye doctor that laser angle treatment frequently stops working and that is why they should have either drops or surgery. In fact, every glaucoma treatment sometimes stops working after a period of control. This can be because the disease gets worse and the baseline pressure is rising, making it look like the treatment has become less effective. But, this is not only true of laser treatment, nor is it likely worse for laser than for eye drops or surgery.

In all the years it's been used, no one has succeeded in making the laser treatment of the angle more effective—despite using a variety of lasers and delivery methods. During the last 10 years, another laser was proposed to be an improvement. This is called selective laser trabeculoplasty or SLT, since its laser energy was delivered over a wider area and at lower power. The claim that one could use this approach repeatedly has been stated, but not proven in any peer-reviewed controlled study directly compared to the established ALT-type laser method. In fact, the existing ALT approach was shown in the past to have some ability to be repeated if it had worked for some years and then the eye pressure rose again. There is no reason to think that the SLT instrument's treatment is either better or worse than the ALT form.

Glaucoma surgery: Until recently, few eye doctors would recommend glaucoma surgery as initial treatment. The general principle of such surgery is to let aqueous humor leak out of the eye through a hole created at the junction of the colored and white part (where the iris meets the sclera) under the covering layer called the conjunctiva. The chief reason to avoid surgery was pretty obvious and often expressed in plain English by patients: "you can't go blind from eye drops, but you can with surgery". As surgery complications decreased over the years, and as we recognized that patients preferred the idea of eye drops, but didn't take them at an ideal rate, some argued that surgery first had a strong argument in its favor.

A large controlled study (the Collaborative Initial Glaucoma Treatment Study) then randomly assigned volunteer, new open angle glaucoma patients to take either eye drops or have trabeculectomy glaucoma surgery (see **Operations for glaucoma**). Ten years into the study, both groups were doing well, and those who got surgery in both eyes were, if anything doing slightly better at preserving their visual field test results. Indeed, as shown in other studies, one can get the eye pressure to fall really low with trabeculectomy. But, 20% of operations had failed within the first year. And as with drops and laser, a small percentage of early successes lose pressure control every year that we follow the patient.

The risks of surgery can be generally grouped into the bothersome and the dangerous. Among the former, patients who have the surgery have minor to modest feelings on the eye that are like a gritty sensation or a feeling as if something is in the eye off and on. Most often these get better quickly. For 1-2% of patients, the feeling in the surgical area is too troublesome and revision surgery is done to relieve it. More serious problems include developing so low an eye pressure that vision is poor, requiring revision surgery to raise pressure. Infections happen early after surgery in one per thousand eyes, and over time, there is a continued chance that the area of surgery makes the eye more susceptible to later infection requiring intensive treatment, revision surgery, and rarely, severe vision loss. Cataract (hazy lens) occurs more often after glaucoma surgery. In fact, there is evidence that all of the glaucoma treatments speed up the development of cataract. While this is undesirable, cataract is surgically removable.

At present, more patients choose eye drops than laser or surgery as their first glaucoma treatment. Yet, a recent large study found that those with serious glaucoma damage did as well or better with first surgery than the comparison group who took eye drops first. Patients who find surgery to be a good first choice are people who can tolerate a bit higher risk, as well as those who feel that they are generally not good at remembering to take medication. Surgery is a good option, then, for those who would like to have the treatment that most allows them to "forget about" their glaucoma.

What is the target pressure?

TAKE HOME POINTS:

- **Making the eye pressure normal is not good enough for many persons**
- **The damaging pressure is assumed to be the present untreated level**
- **It is best to measure the untreated baseline pressure more than once**
- **A pressure about 20-25% lower is the most common initial target**
- **Target should be lower if damage is greater or risk is higher**
- **Both average pressure and how much pressure fluctuates are important**
- **Every patient should have a target pressure**

What is the goal of glaucoma treatment? It is to help persons retain all the useful vision possible for the remainder of their lives without badly bothering them by treatment. In general, we succeed at this with the vast majority of patients. During the descriptions of open angle glaucoma, we mentioned that it is not a disease of elevated pressure in half of those with the disease. So, if your pressure starts out normal and that's the dangerous level for you, it wouldn't help to normalize the pressure, would it? In a very important clinical trial (the Collaborative Normal Tension Glaucoma Study), persons with open angle glaucoma and normal baseline pressure before treatment were randomly given either no pressure lowering, or their pressure was lowered by 30% by drops, laser or surgery. Another key study (the Early Manifest Glaucoma Study) assigned people with untreated glaucoma (many of whom started with normal pressures) to either no therapy or a combination of drops and a laser treatment. The pressures fell in the treated group by about 25% from their untreated level. Both studies showed a real benefit by lowering from a normal pressure level to a lower pressure within the normal range.

It may seem amazing that prior to that last 2 decades, doctors thought that making the pressure normal was successful treatment. In fact, many published studies report that they were successful at treating glaucoma when the pressure was reduced below 21 millimeters of mercury (the upper limit in persons who don't have glaucoma). This was true whether the baseline pressure was 22 or 35! Lowering eye pressure is essential to prevent glaucoma damage. How can we possibly tell how we're doing if we don't have a meaningful goal? Remember that the final outcome that we want to have is to keep useful vision—so it is the visual field test results over time that are the final measure of how you're doing. We do that, but it takes several years to know whether the field test is stable or not. In the mean time, we need a substitute measurement that tells us how we are doing. That's where the target pressure comes in.

Given the results of the major clinical research studies, lowering the pressure by at least 20-25% is a pretty good general target zone. But what was the initial level? Say you go to a new eye doctor and on that visit it is determined that you have open angle glaucoma. To set a target range for treatment by drops, laser or surgery, we need to know the range of pressure that caused the glaucoma damage that has been damaging your optic nerve head or visual field. It could be in the so-called normal range, or it could be higher. Yet, I have seen hundreds of patients put on drops at that first visit with only that one pressure taken. If you're going to be on drops for the rest of your life (or undergoing a procedure for pressure), you should have a good idea of what the starting pressure is. No one likes extra visits to the doctor, but we don't want to rely on only one pressure reading before treatment begins to determine the treatment goal for the next 15 years. We ask patients to come back in 2 more times before starting treatment. We start the therapy on the third visit. Three examples of what happens when we do this are shown in Figure 19. It shows recordings from 3 patients in whom we wanted to start treatment and whose first day pressure was 25. After 3 measurements, the first patient's average was really 25, the second one was usually lower than that (averaging 21), and the third had an average untreated pressure of 30. Without the extra measurements, we'd never know. Eye pressure fluctuates day to day, and fluctuates even more in glaucoma patients. A target set by lowering things 20% in these 3 comes to 3 different pressures when we have a better idea of the baseline.

Can we judge the baseline IOP with only 1 visit?

Visit #1	Visit #2	Visit #3	**Baseline**	**Target**
25	26	25	25	*20*
25	20	18	21	*17*
25	30	35	30	*25*

Figure 19: An illustration of baseline eye pressure determination by making 3 visits in 3 different patients. The average baseline, untreated pressure was the same in each person (25) but after 3 visits, the true baseline was very different among the 3 persons. The target range set for each patient is lower than their baseline by 20%.

I have been asked whether there's a lower limit to the target we set. Can it get too low? For most patients the target is never lower than 12 and for most eyes, 12 is a never too low. It's true that surgery can lower the pressure so low it leads to blurred vision (when it gets below 5 or so). Interestingly, there are lots of eyes than can have a pressure of between 4 and 6 for years and see just fine, while others at this low level are in trouble. We recently looked at 750 eyes in which we had set a target and found that there were 3 main groups, centered at 18, 15 and 12.

The initial drops versus initial surgery study (Collaborative Initial Glaucoma Treatment Study) had a more detailed approach to how much the pressure should be lowered. For those with very early damage, the target lowering was about 20% lower than baseline. Those with bad damage had a target 40% below baseline. Many glaucoma specialists use the general idea that your target needs to be lower if you have more advanced disease. The concept is based on the idea that since we can't get back what is lost, the person with serious damage has less remaining reserve. We don't want to guess too high about where the pressure should have been, since this patient has higher stakes from any further loss.

One approach to determining if the target is achieved when starting eye drops is to use one eye as a comparison for the other. In general, your two eyes have similar variation in their pressures. While it is not perfect, the correlation is far above random, so if pressure goes from lower to higher in the right eye between visits, it will often go in the same direction in the other eye. If we start a new eye drop in the right eye and leave the left temporarily untreated, we can get a decent idea of what the drop did to pressure by comparing the right before and after drops with the untreated left eye on the two visits. This also gives us a good idea of whether any new symptoms might be side effects of the drop, since they would usually only happen in the right eye. But, eyes don't exactly move up and down together, so we will often keep the single-eye trial going for another visit or two to see for sure that the drop achieved the target level. Then, we try it in the second eye. There's no guarantee that the two eyes will behave identically, but in general they do. In some patients, the single-eye trial is not appropriate, and eye drops are started in both eyes.

Most often, working at a referral center, persons coming to us are already receiving treatment prescribed elsewhere. Some of these people have been taking the same drops for 10 years. I often recommend that we find out whether the drops are still "working" by stopping them in one eye for a short time. This is called a unilateral stop trial. This is perfectly safe to do for a short time like a week, since glaucoma doesn't damage eyes in that short a time. And, if you're going to take drops for 10 years or more, it makes sense to see if they're doing anything. I admire and understand patients who are reluctant to do this. They have taken seriously the concept that they must always take their drops. But, the stop trial can help to fix important problems. Imagine that eye pressure fluctuates up and down and that drops are holding it down, but not completely eliminating the variation. You roll along seeing the doctor for 2 or 3 years. Then, on the next visit, the pressure is higher than the target. It might be that you forgot the drops that day. It might be that the eye just had a bad day (big stress or change in health temporarily can raise eye pressure). Many times, we have seen that this leads doctors to prescribe more drops that very day. If we had resisted the temptation to write the new prescription and just measured again a few days later, we could have confirmed that the new drop was really needed, instead of being unnecessary. In past studies, we have found a substantial number of patients are prescribed more drops than they need, probably due to this sequence of events.

We must take pressure fluctuation above the target very seriously, especially if it happens more than once. Recent research has shown that it may be as bad to have a pressure that is varying a lot as it is to have a pressure that on average is above the target. Swings in pressure could have bad effects on the stress generated in the eye wall and on blood flow and ganglion cells. One of the areas that some have studied is how the pressure behaves at night. We all have variations in our body functions from day to night. Our hormone levels follow the sun and moon, and our blood pressure and our eye pressure vary at night compared to daytime. At this time, there are no practical recommendations that have been proven to tell us that pressure measured at night is more important than that measured in the daytime. Some doctors feel that measuring pressure through the course on one day at the hospital is a worthwhile indication of how the patient is doing. There is presently not enough strong evidence that this helps to justify doing it routinely.

We sometimes change the target upwards or downwards. If a patient with glaucoma has done very well over a period of years, we may have set the target pressure lower than it really needs to be. We can then try a higher target level with careful monitoring of the visual field tests for a period of 2 years. On the other hand, we may find that a patient is getting worse in the visual field or optic nerve head structure at the set target level. That means that we have to lower the target range—typically by another 20% compared to the original target—as well as making sure that the patient is truly adhering to the treatment between visits.

Among glaucoma specialists, there are some very good doctors who claim that the target pressure idea is not really needed. I find these arguments difficult to understand. We need to know what we're doing and the idea behind our present target setting is based on very good clinical research. We may not know the exact best target for every glaucoma patient, but every glaucoma patient should have a target pressure to guide the short-term and medium-term treatment, as we look for longer-term stability or worsening in the visual field test.

How to succeed at eye drop treatment: It's all in your hands

TAKE HOME POINTS:

- **The average patient only takes 70% of their drops—don't be average**
- **The chief problem is forgetting, and you don't know you forgot**
- **Using memory aids can dramatically improve drop taking**
- **Link the drops to something else you do, keep them out in plain sight**
- **Follow the 13 tips for taking drops**

Your ability to put a drop on the eye every day means that you are in charge of keeping your vision with glaucoma. But, as we'll see, the secrets of succeeding with drops are as much your head and your wallet as they are in how well you do with the mechanics of eye drop taking. In the next section, we'll talk about the specific medicines now available as glaucoma drops (**Glaucoma eye drops: choices, choices**). Here, we'll talk about how to get the drop in your eye and how to remember to do it.

The dirty little secret of glaucoma drops (until recently) was similar to what used to be a humorous description of the Soviet Russian economy, where salaries were low and no one really did much work.

The joke by Soviet workers was: "I pretend to work and they pretend to pay me". For glaucoma, it was: "I pretend that I take all my drops and the doctor acts like I take them all". Twenty-five years ago, researchers put an early computer in an eye drop bottle and found that patients were taking only 3 out of 4 of their drops—even when the bottles were handed out free.

Studies done in the last 5 years by our Wilmer Glaucoma Center of Excellence have confirmed that little has changed. What we know is very disturbing:

- Of patients who are given a new prescription for glaucoma drops, 25% never fill the second one after getting their first bottle. They had not stopped because the doctor had switched them to another drop).
- Of those who fill the second prescription, only half of all the patients are still taking their drops regularly at the end of the first year (Figure 20). This includes those who switched or went on to surgery or something else.

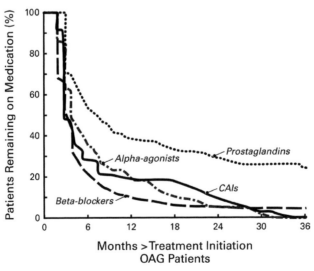

Figure 20: A graph showing that many patients stop refilling prescriptions for their glaucoma drops over time. By one year, less than half were still on drops. Some types of drops had better persistence with drop taking than others.

114

We gave our own patients free glaucoma drops and told them we were going to monitor how many drops they took using an electronic counter on their bottle that recorded when they took the drops. Even though we told them we were keeping track of when they took the drops and urged them to do their best to take them every day, the average patient took only 70% of the drops. Amazingly, when we interviewed these folks and asked how many drops they thought they were taking, they said they were taking 95% or more. I know and respect these patients and I suspect that they believe that they are taking all the drops. So it isn't that they are lying to me. Most of them just don't know that they missed the drops—that's why we call it forgetting. Now with pills, if you have 31 pills to take in a month, when you get to the end of the month and there are 5 pills left, you know you screwed up. With eye drop bottles there's no such clue. If you don't have an iron-clad reminder system, you will forget.

While it isn't an excuse, patients taking pills for long term diseases that have no symptoms (like high blood pressure) do just as badly as glaucoma patients at remembering to take their meds. There's only one kind of chronic medication that does far better than this, where patients take 100% of the pills on time. It's the erectile dysfunction drugs (no surprise there).

Some of our patients took only 20% of the drops. These folks with big adherence problems have some characteristics we can identify. They may have serious memory issues, such as dementia. They may not understand that the drops must go in every day, which means there was a lack of appropriate education. They may have a personality that allows them to ignore that glaucoma can blind you. This is called denial. They do not have a family member with glaucoma. They aren't as likely to have taken the time to find out about glaucoma. By reading this you're marking yourself as someone who is more likely to win by taking drops better. Congratulations! But, if two or more of the statements above apply to you, you may have more trouble remembering drops than you think.

Patients do best with drops right after the doctor visit, tail off between visits, then start using them better again during the week coming up to the visit. We all floss and brush our teeth like mad just before seeing the dentist, so this behavior is understandable though unfortunate. The secret to preventing vision loss is to be consistent and to take drops every day in between visits. As we'll see below, the key to making this happen is to use memory aids that are as strong every day as that just before going to see the doctor feeling.

One of the surprises of our studies was that we thought eye drop side effects were a big cause of not taking drops properly. We found just the opposite! Those who reported redness or stinging or blurring from drops were more likely to be taking them. We should have realized that if you're not taking drops very often, you won't have any side effects. Not that the side effects are that bad—after all, those who reported some minor side effects from drops were taking 9 out of 10 drops dutifully.

So, how can we help patients do better with their drops? Our group has done two big studies that show that effective memory aids work very well. Those who were using only half of their drops improved dramatically after we helped them to do a better job. We tried several ways to remind them. First, we used an alarm that beeped when it was time for the drops. Second, we used telephone calls, emails or text messages at the time that they were supposed to take the drop. These simple efforts helped patients succeed in controlling their glaucoma.

There are some simple memory aids that you can use to help you take all the drops as prescribed. Inexpensive wrist watches can be set to have their alarm go off every day or every 12 hours. Partners and spouses can remind you to take drops. We call this acceptable nagging. A paper calendar sheet and a pencil can be set next to the drop bottle. Every time the drop is taken an X is put on the paper. By checking at the end of month, patients can see when they're forgetting. An example is the patient who found that no drops were getting in every Wednesday night. Wednesday was bridge club night and she came home late and was missing the drops. Anything that changes your usual daily routine will be likely to cause you to forget your drops.

MEMORY AIDS TO REMEMBER DROPS

- **Link drop time to something else you always do**
- **Alarm clock or wrist watch alarm set for eye drop time**
- **Spouse or family member who reminds you every day**
- **Paper calendar sheet and pencil to mark when drops are taken**
- **Taking extra care to remember drops when away from home**
- **Don't hide the bottles in refrigerator or medicine cabinet**

It also matters what time of day the drops are supposed to be used. Patients who plan to take drops every night at bedtime should not get into bed and start reading or watching T.V. before their drops go in, because they are likely to fall asleep and forget to take the drops. Make sure you take the drop whenever you do something you always do, like taking a morning pill, shaving, or putting the coffee pot on to brew. Out of sight, out of mind: don't put drops in the refrigerator or the medicine cabinet. The prostaglandin drops do NOT need refrigeration (see **Glaucoma eye drops: choices, choices**).

The doctor should be part of the solution (and our studies show that some doctors are part of the failure to achieve perfect drop taking). When we studied the behavior of eye doctors with their glaucoma patients, we found they could be grouped into 3 camps, which we called skeptics, reactives, and idealists. The skeptics simply wrote the prescription for drops and acted as if it was up to the patient to take it. When their patients didn't take drops well, they felt that there was nothing that could be done. The reactive group of doctors was willing to try to help patients with adherence with treatment when it was pretty obvious that there was trouble. The final group is one that we hope will be emulated by young doctors in training. These were the idealists—and actual data shows that their patients take their drops better.

Idealist doctors realize that taking medicine is a shared activity between doctor and patient. They establish a non-judgmental environment. For example, they discuss with patients how hard it is to remember to take every drop and agree that it is only human to forget sometimes. They ask questions in an open-ended way that lets patients talk about the problems that they're having. They listen. The skeptic-type and reactive-type doctors in our studies did most of the talking during video-taped study of actual glaucoma visits. They asked closed questions like: "you're taking your drops, right?" for which patients would have to be pretty bold to say "No". Ideal doctors give patients a chance to tell them what they do and don't know about glaucoma. We did a study in which we asked veteran glaucoma patients to tell us what the drops were intended to do. Unfortunately, there were some who didn't understand that drops lower eye pressure and that lowering pressure stopped vision from getting worse. It is too often that we hear: "I'm taking the drops, doctor, but my vision doesn't seem to be getting better". That means we haven't properly educated our patients on how glaucoma treatment stops further damage, but does not restore vision. Finally, ideal doctor behavior is to prescribe only the amount of drops needed, and to keep it as simple as possible.

It's hard enough to remember to take the drops, but using the drops effectively requires more thought than most people realize. Information about drop-taking is unfortunately based on very little scientific data, and pharmacies and drug companies (despite what should be the case) don't always help you to use the right amount of drug efficiently. If you sell a product by the bottle, then having someone use it up as fast as possible makes more money. To paraphrase Winston Churchill, capitalism is the worst form of economic system, except for all the others. We don't have to feel sorry for drug companies and drug store chains—they're making nice profits. But, if you ever had drops come pouring out of a bottle as soon as you began tipping it up toward your eye, you realize that the bottles aren't designed to be easy to use (at least some aren't).

Here are the Lucky 13 ways you can get glaucoma eye drops into the eye and not on the floor, while being effective at lowering eye pressure (and saving money). See Figures 21 and 22 for illustrations.

1. Face the ceiling when putting drops in. Maybe teenagers can look in a mirror, tilt their head way back and get a drop in the eye, but for most of us, several drops wind up on the floor that way. Get horizontal when taking drops, tilt your head way back while sitting in a big comfy chair or better, lie flat in bed.
2. Brace the back of the hand with the bottle on your forehead before tipping it up. We all have tremors and having the bottle waving around without support hurts your aim.
3. Next, before you tilt the bottle over, look up to see that the tip is over the nose half of your eye. Since you're going to be looking through the top of your head (see below) when the drop falls, you can't (and don't want to) see it falling anyway. If any of the drop falls on the area on the nose side of the eye, even if some hits the edge of the eyelid or the inner corner, enough will get on the eye surface to do the job. If you miss on the temple side, it's likely to treat the glaucoma in your ear, not your eye.
4. Pull down the lower eyelid of the eye with the hand that isn't holding the bottle. This increases the target on the white part of the eye. As soon as the drop hits the eye, you can let go.

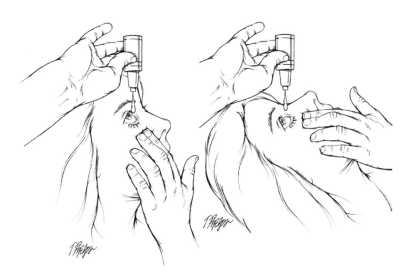

Figure 21: Illustrations of bad drop taking (left) and good drop taking (right). See text for detailed descriptions.

5. Let the bottle deliver as you tip it over and only squeeze if it doesn't come out by itself. This means that you will tip the bottle over, above the nose side of the eye, and let it fall by gravity from about 2 inches or less. Some bottles start having drops come out right away. If the drop doesn't come out by itself, squeeze gently until it does.

6. Use only one drop per eye! Yes, I know that some bottles say put in 2 drops (so does the information sheet from some drug stores). That's a huge waste. Each drop (which has from 25-50 microliters of fluid) contains probably 5 times more drug than is needed for each treatment. So even if you have 80% of it go somewhere else than on the eye surface, you're OK. The drop is absorbed mostly through the clear part of the eye, the cornea. Furthermore, using two drops gives you a greater chance for bad effects on the rest of the body. When you put medicine on the eye, it mixes with the tears, and this drains into the nose through the lacrimal (tear) system in the corner of the eye near the nose. That's why you sometimes taste drops in your nose and throat when you take them. It's also why cocaine abusers snort drug up their nose—it's an effective method to get drugs into the body and head. The same goes for eye drops, but with drops you want the least amount anywhere else other than on the front of the eye.

7. As soon as you hit the eye with drop, close the eyelids and don't blink for 60 seconds. We're now onto some pretty thin ice, scientifically. There is some evidence that not blinking leaves the drop on the eye longer—thus making it go into the eye more. But, when we tested the actual pressure lowering with and without the don't blink instruction, it didn't make a substantial difference. So it makes sense not to blink, but we can't say it has definitive support.

8. Many doctors teach patients to push on the inner nose for 1 minute after putting the drop on the eye, to block the lacrimal drain area and keep drops out of the nose, throat and the rest of the body. Certainly, this naso-lacrimal occlusion makes logical sense, and there is evidence that for children this can reduce the level of drug that can be found in the blood stream

after drops—which is a really good idea if you are someone sensitive to the general body effects of whichever drop you are using. However, very few of my patients are doing nasolacrimal occlusion correctly when I ask them to show me where they're pushing. The fingers must be far back from the bridge of the nose (almost poking the eye) and pushing almost hard enough to hurt in order to stop drug from going to the nose.

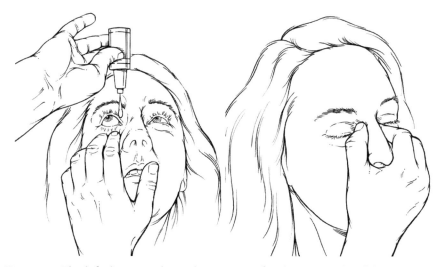

Figure 22: The left drawing shows how to aim for the nose side of the eye to help to get drops in with one drop only. This picture is drawn as if looking down from the ceiling, since your face should be aimed at the ceiling when doing drops properly (see Figure 21). Right drawing illustrates where the fingers are placed to do nasolacrimal occlusion to keep eye drops from going into the nose, throat and rest of the body.

9. After the drop hits and you close your eyes, some will be on the skin of the eyelids. Blot off the excess, since some of us are sensitive to it or may have an actual allergy to the drug or its component parts. We don't want to expose the skin daily to something that may lead to itching, redness, and puffy lids. This requires having facial tissues around before you start putting in drops.

10. You can treat one eye at a time, close, blot, push the nose, and then treat the other eye in the same way. Or, if you're a veteran and can hit both eyes pretty quickly, you can do drop right, drop left and close both, blot both, and push on both sides of the inner nose with the thumb and forefinger for the 60 seconds. If you need to take more than one kind of drop at that time of day, it's faster to do both eyes at once.

11. Wait between two types of drop on the same eye. Many glaucoma patients need to use more than one drug to keep pressure at target. They may have two or three bottles to put in, morning and evening. If you put in drop 1 and in less than 60 seconds you put in drop 2, the second one will wash away the first one and you're not getting the full effect of either one. Now the controversy: how long to wait between bottles? I've heard doctors tell patients to wait 15 minutes! This would mean that the person with 3 kinds of drops would need nearly an hour to get the medicine in. There are no conclusive studies of how long to wait. I suggest that the shortest possible time should be 2 minutes, and if you have a system that lets you wait 5 minutes it's possibly better. However, humans being humans, I know that if you put in drop 1, then say—I'll just dry the dishes and come back for the second drop, you're more likely than not to forget to come back. Don't walk away until they're all in.

12. If you're using more than one type of drop, the order in which they go in doesn't matter. At least something is easy.

13. Running out of medicine can be a big cause of non-adherence. Many pharmacy plans give you either a 1 month or a 3 month supply of drug. They don't usually give you more than you need and typically it is just barely enough if you use one drop at a time. The biggest cause of running out of drug is using too much each time. Use one drop if possible! A second cause for running out is not planning ahead. If you're going to the beach, you won't forget the beach chairs, but an astonishing number of people leave their eye drops at home. Most doctors can fill a new bottle at the ocean-side drug store,

but you'll probably pay full price for it. There is a third rule of drops, namely, they always run out late on Friday night after the doctor's office is closed. Give things a shake on Thursday and see if you're going to need more. Fourth, the Food and Drug Administration (FDA) puts an "expiration date" on drop bottles. This is something to look for when the druggist gives you a 3 month supply—make sure they won't already have expired before the 3 months is up. Finally, a very disturbing (but understandable) finding in one research project was that needing to use a second eye drop type every day led some patients to delay refilling the first bottle until they needed to get both bottles filled. Some drops come as combinations of two types in one bottle and this may help you with this problem

TAKE HOME POINTS: 13 TIPS FOR TAKING EYE DROPS EFFECTIVELY

1. **Face the ceiling**
2. **Brace the back of the hand with the bottle on your forehead**
3. **Look up to see that the tip is over the nose half of your eye**
4. **Pull down the lower eyelid**
5. **Let the bottle deliver by itself**
6. **Use only one drop per eye!**
7. **Don't blink for 60 seconds**
8. **Push on the inner nose: nasolacrimal occlusion**
9. **Blot off the excess**
10. **You can treat one eye at a time**
11. **Wait between two types of drop**
12. **The order in which two drop types go in doesn't matter**
13. **Running out can be a big cause of non-adherence**

Some final aspects of drop taking. When asked to take them twice a day, patients ask if it has to be exactly 12 hours apart. Ideally, yes—but, practically, of course not. It's good enough to hit it two times, one early in the day and one late in the evening. Peg it to something you do at each time, and when you finish the morning dose, and will take the night dose at bedtime, move the bottle to where you'll see it at night (and back after the night dose to where you do the morning dose, if that's a different place). It is totally wrong, however, to take twice a day drops at 9 am and 10 am. Space it out as close to 12 hours apart as much as possible.

Some drops were approved by the FDA to be taken 3 times per day. In desperate circumstances I have patients who do this. They have to think up elaborate schemes for how they're going to take the bottles along wherever they are and how to remember in the middle of a busy day to take them. Generally, I'd rather think of a different way to manage their glaucoma.

Glaucoma eye drops: choices, choices

TAKE HOME POINTS

TAKE HOME POINTS:

- **Prostaglandin eye drops are often selected first because they work best, are convenient and have few side effects**
- **Beta blocker eye drops are often next, sometimes once per day**
- **Twice daily drops, using two different kinds that work together is typically the next step**
- **Generics may save money, but they are not as well tested**
- **The preservative chemical in the drop solution may have big effects, good and bad**

In the preceding section, we dealt with the general issue of taking eyedrops. This section will deal with the individual drop types: which might be better for you, in what order, their strengths and weaknesses, the brand names and generics, and the elephant in the room: cost.

Who's the FDA and why do you care?

The Food and Drug Administration is a government agency that lists its purpose as "protecting the public health by assuring the safety, effectiveness, and security of human and veterinary drugs, vaccines and other biological products, medical devices". Any eye drop that needs a prescription and any device that is used during surgery to lower eye pressure has been checked by the FDA committees and certified. Here's the process as outlined in their web site: Drug companies seeking approval to sell a drug in the United States must test it. First, the drug company or sponsor performs laboratory and animal tests to discover how the drug works and whether it's likely to be safe and work well in humans. Next, a series of tests in humans is begun to determine whether the drug is safe when used to treat a disease and whether it provides a real health benefit. The company then sends the data to the FDA's Center for Drug Evaluation and Research (CDER) to review if the drug is safe and effective for its intended use. A team of CDER physicians, statisticians, chemists, pharmacologists, and other scientists reviews the company's data and proposed labeling. If this review establishes that a drug's health benefits outweigh its known risks, the drug is approved for sale.

Patients often point out to me that they can get "great drugs" in Europe when they visit relatives, or from Asian countries. Some areas of the world have similarly rigorous safety and standardization systems as in the U.S. Some not so much. When studies were done of prostaglandin drugs sold in India, some contained the drug, others didn't, and often the amount wasn't what the label said. The same was true for beta blocker eye drops sold outside the U.S.A. Our approval and oversight system may be slower than elsewhere, but it makes it more likely that you are receiving what you pay for and that drugs have been tested to be safe and effective.

When drug companies develop a new drug, they get a patent to be the only ones to sell it for several years. After the patent ends, theoretically anyone can make the product as a generic drug. The usual reason they do this is to sell it in competition with the brand name drug at a lower price. Generic drugs are approved by the FDA in a less detailed way than the brand name (under patent) drug. The generic maker must present data to show it has the same identity, strength, quality, purity and bioequivalence as the brand name drug. However, for eye drops that does not necessarily mean that the generic was tested on human eyes to see if it lowers IOP as well as the brand, nor that the slightly different formulation used in the generic eye drop won't lead to different side effects. In general, generic drugs do pretty well. One recent study of 38 generic heart pills found them to be fine compared to name brands. Part of the reason is that the brand name company usually produces a generic, too, as soon as the patent runs out—they figure they'll make some of the money in the lower price market, too.

It is left to academic groups like our Center of Excellence to test generic eye drops (at our own expense) or to follow closely what happens to patients who switch to generics. Your drug plan may try to switch you, they may demand that the doctor state that you can only use the brand name, or they may offer the brand name at a higher cost to you. I am unaware of a really bad outcome for the large groups of glaucoma patients that have switched to generic beta blockers, carbonic anhydrase inhibitors, or alpha agonists during the last 10 years. There are patients who firmly want to stay with the brand name they have been using. There's nothing wrong with continuing the brand name, if you can afford it.

Prostaglandins

The first type of eyedrop used by most glaucoma patients is the group called prostaglandins: bimatoprost (Lumigan), latanoprost (Xalatan), and travoprost (Travatan Z). Through this section, we'll use the small letter name for the chemical or generic product and Capital letter for the brand name. The first member of this group to be approved, Xalatan, has been used for over 10 years. As a group, the prostaglandins have the advantages that they only need to be put in once per day and are as effective (or more so) than any of the other drugs that most often need doses both morning and night.

The prostaglandin drugs are close in structure to a natural body chemical found throughout the body. Their discovery as the best glaucoma drug was due to the brilliance and persistence of the late Dr. Carl Camras, who endured years of being told that it wouldn't work. Not long after Xalatan, the other two products (Lumigan and Travatan Z) were approved, and it is fair to say that they are so close to Xalatan that they are essentially the same chemical once they enter the eye. In one large, masked clinical trial, the pressure lowering power of all 3 products was the same and more than 90% of patients who took all 3 drops in sequence found them to have acceptable tolerability. However, Xalatan had significantly fewer patients among the small number who complained of red eyes or some other irritation.

The form of the chemical in Xalatan breaks down more easily and becomes ineffective quicker than the other two. As a result, its bottles have only 2.5 milliliters of fluid in a 5 milliliter bottle. Patients often complain that their bottle was filled only half full and they were cheated. Sorry, but that's done on purpose so that you won't wind up using drops that have no good drug left in them. It's also why the plastic in the Xalatan bottle is so soft—they found that the drug became less effective in standard hard plastic bottles. Newer generic forms of Xalatan (latanoprost) will be marketed soon. The other prostaglandin brand drugs aren't so likely to degenerate, so they can be sold in bigger bottles. But, the trade-off is that they have a greater chance to cause side effects like redness and stinging (there's no free lunch).

The prostaglandin in Travatan Z was recently put into a new vehicle. For any drug, the vehicle has several parts: the drug, the preservative to keep bacteria from growing in the bottle, and chemicals added to prolong the drug life, keep it at the right acidity, and make it more comfortable on the eye. We're paying more attention to the preservative issue now, since there is a lot of evidence that patients sometimes stop being able to tolerate drops because of irritation or allergy caused by the preservative, not the drug in the bottle. For many years, most eye drops used the preservative called benzalkonium chloride, which kills bacteria well, and even helps to

128

get the drop into the eye better. But, if you became allergic to ben-zalkonium, you were in trouble, as most of the drops had it—so you couldn't take any of them. More recently, every class of glaucoma drug has an alternative brand with different preservative, and one can obtain preservative-free versions of some drugs at significantly increased cost.

The side effects from a drug can be listed in various ways. In this section, I'm going to distinguish between what I call the possible side effects and all the others that are listed by the FDA paper that comes with drugs or the lists that are handed out by drug stores, chains, and prescription plans. The possible side effects are things that happen often enough that you might actually have them hap-pen to you. They are side effects that are clearly associated with taking the drop type based on good evidence. These go away when the drug is stopped and come back when it is restarted. This doesn't mean that a unique side effect couldn't happen just to you and not to anyone else. Our approach at the Glaucoma Center of Excellence is always to stop a drop when a patient thinks something bad is due to the medicine. We like to see if the side effect comes back when the drug is restarted, too. While it is reasonable to always suspect the drug, it's easy to test whether the drug is the cause by this type of stop trial.

The long lists of side effects that are listed for each drug by the FDA, and sometimes handed out by drug stores, contain side effects that rare and even ones that actually aren't related to the drug. Drugs are tested for effectiveness by comparing the response of people treated with the drug to people who took drops that haven't got any drug in them. These dummy drops are called placebos, and we use them to show that the drug has a real effect that wouldn't be seen by chance. The FDA listing includes as a side effect anything that happened to 1 in 100 (1%) or more persons in the year-long studies done to get the drug approved. However, they include things that happened 1% of the time whether they happened in the drug-treated group or the placebo group. So, prostaglandin eye drops are said to be more likely to cause upper respiratory infec-tions, probably because there were a lot of colds in everyone in the final study trial. Prostaglandin eye drops have a tiny amount of chemical per drop. The amount is measured in micrograms, or millionths of a gram. Most of it winds up staying in the eye, or it is broken down before it gets into the blood stream. In fact, I have been told you can't measure any prostaglandin drug in the blood after standard doses. So how could it cause systemic things like a cold? Some of the things I've seen on drug store side effect lists have never happened during my 40 years' experience seeing glaucoma patients every week. The best approach is to ask your doctor about side effects you are worried about.

The possible side effects of prostaglandins are all in the eye. Most common is growing longer and thicker eyelashes. This led to development of a commercial product in mascara brushes that is marketed to grow lashes. In general, it's not so vigorous a growth that the lashes become a problem, and many consider it a nice side effect. Rarely, fine hair can grow on the eyelid skin, or lashes grow in the corner of the eye. In some persons, lashes grow so big that they turn in and rub on the eye. Also, the amount of a pigment called melanin increases with this drop. This is the same pigment that leads to tanning from the sun. That means that the iris and the skin around the eyes can turn a darker color after treatment. For those who tell me that their wife married them "because of my beautiful hazel eyes", having the iris turn browner is sometimes not acceptable. It happens to only a minority of those treated, but it is permanent when it happens to the iris, even when drug is stopped. It is not noticeable if you have brown eyes to start with. Most often, patients tell me that they care if they see with their eyes, not what color their eyes are. The darkening of eyelid skin is reversible if the drug is stopped. These side effects happen to a similar extent with all the brands of prostaglandin.

Other possible effects of prostaglandins are the eyes becoming red, irritated, puffy, or definitely allergic. Allergy shows itself by itching that goes on all day and redness and swelling that often include the eyelid skin. While it does happen with prostaglandins, allergy is infrequent. Finally, there are events that happen in a few unlucky patients, but one can't say for sure that they are actually due to the drug. With the following conditions, it is said that prostaglandins can make the disease occur or reoccur if it was present before: inflammation (uveitis), herpes infections of the cornea, and swelling of the retina (macular edema). Interestingly, in each of these cases, a report was published showing a small group of patients who got the problem, stopped the prostaglandin, and had the condition go way, then got the condition again when given the drug a second time. I've treated hundreds of persons with these conditions who got the benefit of the drug, and didn't have these disorders occur. We discuss this with each patient who has no alternative drug and might be at risk for the side effect before using it, or choosing to move on to other therapy.

How do the prostaglandins lower the eye pressure? It's an interesting story, but to make it short, they work to allow aqueous out of the eye by two ways. Early after their discovery, it was found, in animal eyes, that they change the makeup of the ciliary body at the base of the iris through the uveoscleral outflow pathway, a path that allows aqueous to exit through the space between the choroid and the sclera. There wasn't much attention paid after that to effects of prostaglandins on the more standard trabecular meshwork pathway. But, the mechanism of changing the chemical content of the ciliary body would take days to weeks to happen, and the drug is well-known to lower eye pressure the same day it starts. So, later work has shown that at least one and probably all of the prostaglandins lower pressure also by improving outflow of aqueous through the standard meshwork outflow path.

Beta blockers

Our nervous system has large unconscious components which are very useful. These unconscious components mean you don't have to think about digesting lunch while reading this guide; the autonomic nerves do that for you on autopilot. These systems are controlled by chemicals that work like a lock and key. The chemical that activates the process is the key and the lock into which it fits is its "receptor". When the key is in the lock, things happen. In addition, there are chemicals that fit the lock, but don't activate the mechanism. These are called blockers or inhibitors. The unconscious nervous system has two main parts: the adrenergic and parasympathetic. Adrenergic receptors come in two flavors, given the Greek letters alpha and beta (A and B). Some 40 years ago, it was recognized that molecules that inhibit the beta adrenergic receptors strongly inhibit the making of aqueous humor at the ciliary body. Thus, they are called beta blockers. In the form of pills, millions of persons take this class of drug to lower blood pressure, decrease the chance of another heart attack, treat abnormal heart rhythm, and prevent migraine. Their generic names most often end in –olol (like propranolol).

The first beta blocker eyedrop approved by the FDA in 1978 was timolol (with the brand name Timoptic) which has long since gone generic, and there are now other forms of timolol (Betimol, Istalol, Timoptic XE) as well as related beta blockers like levobunolol (Betagan), betaxolol (Betoptic), and carteolol (Ocupress). The generic agents seem to lower eye pressure as well as the original brands of beta blockers. In some patients there is enough action from these agents that they can be used only once per day, but more frequently they need to be taken morning and night. Timolol's ability to lower pressure is used as the gold standard for how good other drops need to be. There are different strengths (0.25%, 0.5%, and 1%) of some of the beta blockers available.

The possible side effects of beta blockers are both eye problems and general body issues. In the eye, there is tendency for eyes with poor tear function to make fewer tears. This is called dry eye syndrome or keratitis sicca. It is very common that the tears we make don't keep the eye comfortable because they lack the oily components that keep tears from evaporating away too quickly. When little dry spots form, they hurt like needles or sand in the eye. In response, the eye tries to make more tears, but they're as bad as they were before, so now there's a sandy gritty feeling and the eye is tearing. The eye doctor will tell you to help dry, tearing eyes by putting artificial tears on the eye. This sounds wrong, since you've already got tears in your eyes. Think of it as fighting fire with fire: you're fighting tears with better tears. The non-prescription artificial tears have the oily component your own tears lack, so the tearing stops because a more effective, non-evaporating layer is formed by them. None of these tears we're talking about has anything to do with the aqueous humor inside the eye, which never gets out onto the cornea. Tears come from a gland mostly up under the temple side of the upper eyelid. We don't know why beta blocker drops make dry eyes worse, but if you are having symptoms like this, ask the doctor to stop the beta blocker to see if it helps. Allergy to the drug is uncommon with beta blockers, but it happens.

Now as a general rule, any time a patient thinks that a side effect is caused by a drop, consider stopping it immediately for a few days in one eye. That way you can compare the treated to the untreated eye. Often, the symptom isn't helped and we find out the drop isn't the cause. When it is confirmed that the drop is the problem, we find a different one to take. This is the unilateral stop trial mentioned before.

The general body effects of beta blockers (or any drops) come through exposure of the drug to the surfaces inside the nose—the drops get there through the tear drainage system—hence, the description of how to block this with your fingers in the preceding section by nasolacrimal occlusion. All the reasons that beta blocker pills are given to treat disease can be bad side effects in people who are very sensitive to them: very slow heart beat, lowered blood pressure, and intensification of wheezing in people with asthma or chronic lung disease. In fact, beta blocker eyedrops are almost never used in people with asthma. Some of the beta blockers actually raise the blood level of the bad kind of cholesterol. And, in some people there is a psychological depression and a loss of the appetite for sex in men. Naturally, any of these is significant enough that if they are happening due to drops, we change them.

Carbonic anhydrase inhibitors

The system that makes aqueous humor at the ciliary body is driven by a chemical (enzyme) called carbonic anhydrase. In the 1950s, two researchers at the Wilmer Institute (Tom Maren and Bernard Becker) realized that blocking this enzyme chemically would decrease the formation of aqueous and lower eye pressure. For 30 years, we had only a pill to do this with, but more recently the eye drop formulations dorzolamide (Trusopt) and brinzolamide (Azopt) were developed and work almost as well as the pills and without the general body side effects that make acetazolamide (Diamox) and methazolamide (Neptazane) pills so hard for patients to tolerate. The eye drop form has to be used twice per day, and the FDA felt that it really did best when taken 3 times per day when these were the only drops used to lower eye pressure. When patients are taking more than one drop to lower the eye pressure, it is reasonable to use this class of medicines twice a day. The pill forms of this type of medicine are taken from once up to 4 times per day. Generic dorzolamide has been a reasonable substitution for the brand name.

Possible side effects of this group of drops are that they sting more than the other glaucoma drops for minutes after being given. And, in about one in ten patients they leave an unpleasant taste in the mouth, described as metallic. Allergy is about as common as with beta blockers. Fortunately, there have been no reports over the 10 years that these drops cause the general body problems that are caused by the pill forms. These include a severe tiredness, mental depression, pins and needles sensation in the lips and fingers, kidney stones, and worst of all, a form of loss of all blood cells that can be severe in a very small number of persons (aplastic anemia). When we are facing a very serious, acute form of very high pressure, we still prescribe these pills for temporary periods to save vision. Some persons have taken them for years with no problems and for them they remain a good solution.

Alpha agonists

Just as blocking beta adrenergic receptors helps by cutting down aqueous formation, stimulating the other type, alpha receptors, with an agonist helps by speeding water flow out through the uveoscleral pathway, as well as to decrease inflow of aqueous, both combining to lower pressure. There are 3 drugs in this class, only one of which is most commonly used for chronic glaucoma therapy, brimonidine (Alphagan P). Brimonidine both generically and as the brand name Alphagan has come as 0.1%, 0.15% and 0.2%. The companies have tried marketing the lower strengths in the hope that the side effects will be lessened without losing the power to lower pressure. Patients should pay attention to which strength they are getting to keep it consistent, though even experts can't tell any difference in the effects. Generic brimonidine appears a reasonable alternative to the brand.

The drug apraclonidine (Iopidine) was originally approved for very short term use, but is still occasionally used in the same role as brimonidine. Both have as their biggest possible side effect a frequency of allergic reaction that is significantly higher than all other glaucoma drugs. If a patient is taking 4 kinds of drops and develops an allergy, I always stop the alpha agonist first to see if it clears up and 9 times out of 10 that is the drop causing it. Doctors see this reaction as lumps called follicles on the white part of the eye's surface covering, the conjunctiva. This was also characteristic of an older alpha drug, dipivefrin (Propine) and all the prior epinephrine group of eye drops in this class used back in the 1960s. Brimonidine rarely causes people to feel like they have to fall asleep even during the daytime, and it is should never be used in infants or young children. General body reactions that occur with some frequency with brimonidine are a feeling of dryness in the mouth and feeling tired. Theoretically, it could increase heart rate or blood pressure, but this was not found in formal research studies.

There is some evidence that brimonidine has protective effects in glaucoma in addition to its lowering of eye pressure. Brimonidine was tested in humans with different eye disease from glaucoma and there was no apparent benefit to ganglion cells, the nerve cells that die in glaucoma. A recent study in glaucoma patients suggests that it might slow glaucoma damage more than timolol did. Unfortunately, the small number of patients studied and the dropout of more than half the brimonidine patients from side effects makes the study less than powerful as proof that the drug works other than by lowering eye pressure. By law, companies can only claim that a drug works for the reasons shown in experiments that they give to the FDA. Thus, it is not correct to say at this time that brimonidine or any other eye drop protects the eye by any mechanism other than lowering the pressure. The law has not prevented drug salespersons from making unfounded claims for their drugs. They know that if they say something often enough, it becomes what I call "marketing truth". Say it enough, and people believe it is true, even if the evidence isn't there. That is to be different from scientific truth, which requires that objective research be done and show that the claimed benefit is real.

Parasympathomimetics

In the other half of the unconscious nervous system from the alpha and beta sympathetic group, we have the parasympathetic system. The drugs that affect this system work by stimulating little muscles within the eye to contract. One particularly visible result is that they make the pupil small. The one remaining drug in this class still found in drug stores is pilocarpine, which improves outflow of aqueous. It has so many downsides that it is used infrequently, and usually for special situations. It causes blurred vision, dim vision, a sinus-headache-like pain, redness of the eye, and occasionally can cause a detachment of the retina inside the eye. The most common time that eye surgeons still use this class of drug is as a help during the production of a laser iris hole for angle closure (iridotomy), or, as part of cataract surgery to make the pupil smaller.

Osmotic agents

In the middle of a very high pressure emergency, doctors sometimes give medicine that is designed to lower the eye pressure quickly to make other treatment possible. This means drinking a solution containing the drug or receiving it as an infusion into a vein. In both cases, the way it works is to send a big dose of sugar-like chemical through the blood stream. Because the blood is temporarily lower in water content compared to the eye, water is sucked out of the eye into the blood vessels in the choroid and retina. These agents are called glycerol and mannitol. They can only be given under careful observation in a medical facility.

Combinations of drops

In order to make the use of more than one type of drop every day easier, companies have made (so far) combinations of beta blockers with both dorzolamide (dorzolamide—timolol generic, or Cosopt brand name) and with brimonidine (Combigan, brand name only). In general, these have as good an effect in lowering eye pressure as the two drugs in separate bottles. They are most often prescribed two times a day.

Special circumstances with drops

Children can be given eyedrops when they have glaucoma, but we must note that brimonidine—and by extension apraclonidine—were associated with severe sleepiness and possibly coma in young kids. These alpha agents should never be given to children under age 8.

When I meet a young woman with primary or secondary glaucoma who is in the child-bearing years This does happen, though glaucoma is more a disease of the older population. I have a conversation about drugs and pregnancy. While a previous generation of pregnant women possibly took pills and had a nightcap (my Mom did), now we try to avoid any chemical influences on unborn children at all. First, I am not aware of one example of an eye drop that has been shown to cause a birth defect in a child. And, due to having seen a lot of women who didn't tell me they were pregnant until the second or third trimester, I've seen a lot of pretty babies born to Moms who were taking glaucoma drops. But, to plan this most appropriately, if we assume that many couples use contraception, then it only makes sense to plan what to do about your glaucoma drops before stopping contraception. If you wait until the pregnancy test is positive, much of the critical first trimester has already passed and the fetus has already been exposed to the drugs.

3 CHOICES FOR GLAUCOMA TREATMENT IN WOMEN WHO WISH TO BE PREGNANT

1. **Keep going with the drops to protect Mom's eyes, and hope that there are no ill effects**
2. **Stop the drops during pregnancy and breast-feeding and watch Mom's visual field testing closely**
3. **Switch to laser treatment or glaucoma surgery prior to the pregnancy.**

Each of these has been the choice of some patients of mine and their partners, and the decision really must be made on an individual basis. I've seen each to be the best choice for someone. I can say that based on what I know of the drugs, there is no reason to think that one of the eye drop types is safer than the others in this regard.

Laser glaucoma surgery: iris holes and angle treatment

TAKE HOME POINTS:

- Laser iris holes are made in one or both eyes with eye drop anesthesia, as an outpatient
- Iridotomy is pretty painless and usually a permanent hole is made in one sitting
- Iris holes occasionally cause glare and possibly can speed cataract development
- Laser angle treatment is comfortable and highly safe to vision
- Angle treatment whether done over half or whole meshwork has only a modest pressure effect
- ALT and SLT type angle treatment accomplish similar results, with no proof one is better
- Repeat angle treatment can work, but less often than first time treatment

Preceding sections mentioned where laser treatment fits into decision-making in the treatment of open angle glaucoma (**What treatments are the right ones? Drops, scissors, laser**) and angle closure glaucoma (**Why isn't glaucoma either there or not there—what makes you an angle closure suspect?** and **Acute angle closure**

crisis). We will now consider what it's like to go through the procedures, a laser iris hole or laser angle treatment.

Informed consent

Probably every reader has signed an informed consent form for a procedure at some point. Did you read it? Did you have any questions answered? Were you sure that the benefits of the procedure outweighed the risks? For laser interventions and surgical procedures, it is in your best interest to be sure that you did these things before going ahead. Patients will often say to me that they don't want to have a procedure because they are afraid of the complications. That's a very understandable feeling. But, we have two risks to consider: the risk of the procedure and the risk of what may happen to you now from the disease itself if you don't have the procedure. How big are these compared to each other? That's the thing that should make up your mind as to whether to sign and go ahead. It's the doctor's job to explain both risks to you, and to outline the benefits of the procedure (and the benefits of not having it).

For the laser treatments to be considered in this section, the risks are very low, but they are never zero. Listen carefully and ask all the questions you and your family can think of. Write down what you want to ask at home and bring in your list of questions.

Laser iridotomy (iris hole)

The procedure is done as an outpatient and it is best to have someone along to take you home, as your vision in one or both eyes might be poor for driving or walking, though it isn't usually badly blurred. We can treat one or both eyes at one sitting. There is no preparatory medicine needed on the day before or morning of, and you should take any usual eyedrops that were prescribed for daily use. After the preliminary exam, an eye drop of pilocarpine (see **Glaucoma eye drops: choices, choices**) is put into the eye to make the pupil small and the iris thinner. This takes 15-30 minutes. You will get a pressure sensation, often felt in the eyebrow, and your vision can change temporarily. The eye is numbed with anesthetic eye drop or ointment and a lens is put on the eye, held by the doctor's fingers to keep your eyelids out of the way and to magnify the view. You will be sitting up at the instrument called the slit lamp with a chin rest and bright light shining from binoculars that the doctor looks through. You help by keeping the other eye open and staring straight ahead between blinks. It's OK to blink, since the eye getting treated can't close with the examining lens in place.

The most commonly used laser is the neodymium:YAG type, which treats the eye so fast that you won't have a chance to move your eye during laser applications. When the laser fires, you get a sensation that something happened. It's typically not unpleasant, just a little startling if the doctor doesn't warn you first. We often need to make several deliveries of laser to produce a hole about one half a millimeter in size, about the size of a ball point pen tip (Figure 17). That's all it takes to let aqueous flow from behind to in front of the iris and fix the problem. It's pretty uncommon that you or someone else will see where the hole was made, though if you look closely you'll later possibly see a black dot where it is. Because the laser is focused down to a point at the iris inside the eye, it doesn't have concentrated power anywhere in the eye except there, so it doesn't damage the wall of the eye or anything behind the iris. You won't have a hole in the outer wall of the eye.

Among glaucoma specialists there is a controversy about where on the iris the best place for the hole is. It doesn't matter from the point of view of water moving through, since anywhere works. A small number of persons after iridotomy report that they see an additional line of light around street lights, or, they see more glare in general. Some believe that this is because the hole in the iris is right behind where the upper eyelid and its tear film lies, producing an optical effect called light scattering. For this reason, most of us put the hole far up in the peripheral iris, while other doctors claim that it's best to put it right out in the middle of the iris (at 3 or 9 o'clock if the iris were a clock). Most persons find this disturbing optical effect goes away with time, but occasionally an additional treatment is needed to make it go away.

For the first hour after treatment, vision is blurred, but it clears quickly. One hour after treatment the pressure is checked, since occasionally it rises substantially and needs treatment for a while with drops to make it safe again. No eye patch is used. Often, anti-inflammatory eye drops are given 4 times per day for a few days. The next visit is 1 - 6 weeks later. If the laser hole is not open at 6 weeks after the initial treatment, it is retreated, which is typically pretty quick and easy. Making a hole is harder in thicker, brown irises, such as in African- or Asian-derived persons. In them, we sometimes gang up two treatment with two separate types of lasers in sequence, the first being a continuous wave laser (diode) to thin down the iris, followed by the neodymium:YAG to punch through. About one in ten times in this kind of patient it can take two sessions to make a full hole of the right size.

Once a laser iris hole is made, it's pretty much open for good. The iris doesn't heal as do other body tissues, probably because the aqueous fluid that surrounds it contains chemicals that prevent healing under normal circumstances. The exceptions to the no-healing rule are eyes that have new blood vessels growing in them or eyes with inflammatory processes (neovascular and inflammatory glaucoma, see **Secondary glaucoma**). Because the normal situation of no-healing is changed by these processes, laser iris holes in those eyes can close up and are watched more closely.

There is some limited evidence that making a hole in the iris speeds the development of cataract, perhaps because the movement of aqueous is re-routed through the hole and doesn't uniformly bathe the lens as it normally does. Of course, if the eye develops an acute angle closure crisis because the hole wasn't made, a cataract is pretty much guaranteed to develop soon. An iris hole, on balance, may wind up preventing more cataract than it might cause if angle closure (crisis or not) is avoided. The only other serious complication of laser iridotomy was reported many years ago, when an older type of laser was being used and the laser was focused by mistake far into the eye, causing a spot in that eye's vision. This is avoided by careful aiming and focusing and to our knowledge has never happened with the newer laser.

Laser angle treatment (trabeculoplasty: LTP, ALT, or SLT)

As with iridotomy, laser angle treatment is done as an outpatient, one or both eyes can be treated in one sitting, and no pre-operative drugs are needed. You eat and drink normally on the day of treatment. The eye is numbed with drops and an examining lens is put on the eye so you can't close the eye during blinking. The lens has a mirror to let the doctor see the meshwork all around its 360 degree circle as the lens is gradually turned during treatment. The two types of lasers used are the continuous wave laser (argon or diode type for ALT) or the neodymium:YAG laser tuned specially for this treatment (selective laser trabeculoplasty, SLT). ALT has been used since 1978, while the SLT was developed in the early 2000s. The size of the area illuminated by ALT and SLT are different, but from the patient's point of view, there is no real difference, since it is unusual for you to feel anything as 80-100 spots are shined on the meshwork when the entire 360 degrees are treated. The treatment takes less than 10 minutes per eye.

The eye pressure is measured 60 minutes after treatment, no patch is used, and glaucoma drops are continued until 6 weeks or more after treatment, which is how long it takes to see the effect (or not). Eye drops containing anti-inflammatory medicine may be used for a few days at about 4 times per day to decrease redness and discomfort. In thousands of laser angle treatments done at our Institute, I have not seen a person whose vision or health was made worse by the treatment itself. That's a big vote in favor of the small risk of doing laser angle treatment. We simply wish that it had a stronger effect on pressure than it does, and despite much variation in how it is delivered, no one has come up with a more potent method. For people already taking eye drops, only about 2/3 of those treated have a big enough further lowering of pressure to call it helpful. Most are still taking eyedrops afterward. So laser angle treatment is sometimes said to be like "adding another drop".

The way the ALT or SLT works is thought to be by a micro-injury to the trabecular meshwork. Injured tissue puts out chemicals for healing that apparently signal the cells there to behave more normally, dividing into new cells, and making better surrounding material that lets water out faster. Fluid from the juice overlying experimentally treated trabecular meshwork from human eye bank eyes causes untreated meshwork cells to improve their function.

Clearly, we don't want to cause major injury or to injure all of the meshwork badly, or the pressure would go up instead of down. In fact, in my laboratory, we have developed animal models of high eye pressure by extensive lasering of the meshwork. The ALT type treatment affects only 10% of the meshwork directly by its injury, while the SLT pretty much exposes the entire meshwork to energy, but at a lower level. From all present data, the two treatments wind up with the same level of pressure lowering. This means that the level of injury caused by SLT is less per "pound" of meshwork, but it accomplishes the same thing.

Some doctors treat only half of each eye at one sitting of ALT or SLT. The idea is that you can see some lowering from such a treatment and later one could come back and do the other half and get the same effect again. This sounds fine, but the available evidence suggests that treating half the eye gets less effect than treating the whole 360 degrees. If half treatment got a really big effect, it would be a stronger argument for it. Unfortunately, ALT and SLT really only work well to control pressure at the target level by all by themselves about 1/3 of the time. Drops are needed still in the rest, and in 1/3 there is no effect at all. Although it is reasonable to perform only 180 degrees of laser treatment, my view has been that doing a half treatment may not be enough, and by splitting treatments into halves and waiting for effects, we are delaying getting the eye to a safer pressure. I certainly don't feel that dividing the treatment into halves is wrong, however. The other issue is from a cost perspective, doctors charge the full price for a half or a whole treatment, so doing it twice doubles the cost to the health care system (or Medicare, for which we all pay).

Even more controversial is repeated LTP treatment. Some years ago, a case series of patients who had undergone full 360 degree ALT once, and had a good effect for years, were retreated when the effect wore off. About 40% seemed to get another good long effect, but the others didn't. In another such full retreatment study, 10% of the retreated eyes had the pressure go up instead of down, some requiring fairly prompt surgery to lower pressure. When SLT instruments began to be marketed, the makers claimed that it was more repeatable than ALT, and that since its energy levels were lower than ALT, repeat treatment would be better or safer. That's the marketing truth (see **Glaucoma eye drops: choices, choices**), but there has been no study that shows that SLT is more repeatable than we already know ALT is. I have now seen patients who had repeated SLT whose pressure went higher, requiring prompt surgical operations in the operating room to bring it down. The scientific truth is that any laser angle treatment could get a second decrease in pressure from repeat treatment, but it is true for both laser types, and repeat treatment has not only a high failure rate, but a small risk of causing higher pressure.

Operations for glaucoma

TAKE HOME POINTS:

- **Pre-operatively, we review your medical health, present medicines, and allergies**
- **You must consider stopping things that increase bleeding: including aspirin, vitamin E**
- **You won't feel the surgery or be able to see it**
- **A patch will be on the eye for the first night only**
- **Bring someone with you to the surgicenter**
- **Don't eat anything after midnight for surgery the next day**
- **One eye at a time**

The idea that surgery in an operating room is the last resort has been a frequent comment by patients we care for. Certainly in terms of the three main treatments (drops, laser, surgery), the one that could cause vision loss by itself is surgery. This is not very common, but it doesn't help much to tell a person with a surgical complication that it only happens one in 100 times when they are the one. So, in general, patients do select surgery second or third in line as glaucoma treatments. But, remember that the Collaborative Initial Glaucoma Treatment Study found that surgery before anything else was at least as effective in protecting patients from vision loss as drops. It is the approach most likely to result in no need for daily medication. The decision about which of the three main treatment approaches you want to use was considered in section **Which treatments are the right ones: drops, scissors, laser?** Here, we will deal with what patients go through during the various types of glaucoma surgery, why we'd use one over the other one, and what the future holds for procedures that are now being tried out.

The main types of glaucoma surgery are trabeculectomy, tube-shunt surgery, and diode laser ciliodestruction. At the present time, eye surgeons would most often recommend them in that order, with trabeculectomy being far and away the most commonly performed, especially for those who have not had surgery before. Let's consider what you'd go through if you choose glaucoma surgery. Many of the events are similar with the 3 surgery types.

Pre-operatively, you would sign an informed consent form after a discussion, in which it is explained that the benefits of surgery are bigger than the risks, and that the risk of surgery is smaller than the risk you now have from the disease as it is being treated. This is a chance to ask questions and make sure that you understand the process. You will have a brief physical exam and review of your medical health and present pills (we need their real names and doses, not just "a blood pressure pill", so bring along the bottles of medicine). All patients get some form of anesthesia, usually both on the eye itself and in the vein. Some doctors do this themselves with help from a nurse, while in hospitals and many surgicenters, there is a nurse anesthetist or an anesthesiologist present who monitors you during the surgery. The eye doctor and the anesthesia staff need to know if you've had recent health issues that could affect you during eye surgery. It isn't that there are big effects on your heart as you might have in abdominal surgery, but the excitement of surgery can run your blood pressure up or get your heart skipping beats. We also need to assure that we don't give you medicine that you are allergic to, or that would interact badly with your present medicines. Many centers ask you not to eat the morning of surgery, so that in case you get an upset tummy, there's nothing to bring up.

It is particularly important that you stop taking pills that can make you bleed more than we want during eye surgery. This includes aspirin, Coumadin (warfarin), Plavix, heparin, and any multivitamin that contains vitamin E. Some persons need blood thinners because of serious medical conditions like clots in leg veins, atrial fibrillation heart rhythm, or artificial heart valves. In these cases, we have special ways to keep the blood thinning going and do the surgery anyway. But if you're simply taking a baby aspirin or vitamins for good health, stop them as long prior to surgery as possible. Check with your medical doctor first before changing anything.

You'll have a needle placed in a vein, both to give sedative medicine, and to be able to give you drugs in case they're needed. You will have monitoring devices attached to you for your heart rate, blood pressure (the cuff gets tight), and oxygen level in the blood (on a finger clip). You will be flat on your back in a bed-like stretcher during the surgery, which will take less than an hour from coming into the operating room to going back to family. The area around the eye gets prepared in sterile fashion and plastic drapes stick to your face so only the eye is visible to the surgeon. You will not be able to see what is going on during the operation, though quite often you can hear what happens in the room, music, instruments being asked for, and chit chat about my beautiful grandchildren (to distract you pleasantly).

Before starting, our group gives a medicine that puts you to sleep for 5 or 10 minutes intravenously. During the brief time that you are asleep, we numb the whole area around the eyeball with a local anesthetic. You wake up in a few minutes with no feeling around the eye. You can't move your eye, because the eye muscles on that side are paralyzed. An instrument is put in to hold your eye open, so you can't blink the eye that is being worked on. All you have to do is try to relax and generally keep your body still. If you need to move or cough or scratch your nose, or if you're in pain, you can just speak up and you will be taken care of by staff. It's important not to move your arms or legs, and not to talk unless there is pain, since all that causes the eye to move. It's not a good idea to give the microsurgeon a moving target. Some surgeons use less anesthesia, none in the vein, and only eyedrops and little injections near the eye during surgery—the advantage is less chance for bad reaction to medicine, but some patients don't want to be that aware of what's going on. If you get anxious during the surgery, we can give more sedative and narcotics to stop any pain. It is rare, but some extremely anxious patients or others who cannot stay still during surgery, elect to have general anesthesia.

The surgeon is looking at your eye through a binocular microscope hung over the eye aimed down at you. Also watching are one or more surgical assistants, a nurse handing instruments over, a nurse getting things for us, and anesthesia staff. In a teaching institution like ours, there are large plasma screens with your operation shown to those learning in the room. You will hear the surgeon asking assistants to cut things, hold things, and keep things moist. Believe it or not, we often have four different instruments on or in the eye at one time, so it takes a village.

Unlike general surgery, we never need to do blood transfusions for eye surgery. At the conclusion of surgery, you will most often have a patch placed on the eye to protect it for the first night. The local anesthetic blocks vision as well as feeling, so your vision would be pretty bad anyway, and the eye is much more comfortable patched that first 12 hours. It is tricky getting around with only the unpatched eye—your depth perception is gone, so get help on stairs and curbs. Holding hands with someone friendly is a great idea anytime, but especially now.

It's mandatory to bring someone with you to the surgicenter the day of surgery. Hospitals have rules that when you get a sedative you shouldn't go home by yourself. For those having surgery on their better seeing eye, it is obvious that someone will need to help you the night of surgery to do all your essential things, like getting to the bathroom. Overnight admission to the hospital is no longer permitted for standard eye surgery.

For most glaucoma operations, you won't need much pain medicine. Over the counter pain pills will usually keep you comfortable, but remember: nothing containing aspirin until you are told to restart it. The eye will be sore, especially when you look around, due to some bruising. Eyelids get swollen temporarily, and there can be a black eye as a small amount of blood can seep under the skin of the eyelid. Try to make up a better story for friends than walking into a door. The upper eyelid droops some after most surgeries (called ptosis with a silent "p"). Almost always this goes away by itself—and it keeps you more comfortable by covering the eye more as it heals. If it stays too long, a minor outpatient plastic procedure can be done to raise the lid.

You will almost surely not have the same vision right after surgery as right before, but in most cases vision is back to how it was before surgery within 1-2 weeks. The blurring comes partly from microscopic particles of blood and other tissues inside the eye during this time, and unfortunately you're looking through them. Any major worsening of your vision after surgery should be brought to the surgeon's attention right away.

The operation did something to the surface covering of the eye (conjunctiva), often involving small stitches, so you will sometimes have a feeling that something is in the eye. We try to minimize this by making the stitches of really tiny material and material that absorbs on its own. You'll be putting in frequent eyedrops as directed by the surgeon, and these help to smooth over the surface. Some of the drops are anti-inflammatory (they help with redness and swelling), while others are temporary antibiotics.

You will be given a set of written instructions with all the detailed "dos and don'ts" that the surgeon suggests. This will deal with physical activity, bathing habits, and travel. Along with this will be the emergency phone number. It is far better to call and ask a question that you think might be silly than to take a chance that you'll not want to bother the surgeon and let something bad go on too long.

Except in infants, it is very rare for eye surgery to be done in both eyes on the same day.

Trabeculectomy

TAKE HOME POINTS FOR TRABECULECTOMY

- **It works by producing a controlled leak of eye fluid outward**
- **The area of surgery (bleb) is not usually visible except to your closest buddies**

- **The target pressure is reached gradually by releasing stitches, painlessly**
- **Success is achieved for years in the majority of patients**
- **Problem areas are: too low eye pressure, late infection, and cataract**

Some patients want to know every detail of their surgery. So, we have made available videos of glaucoma surgery on the Glaucoma Center of Excellence website. Other patients only want to know the general principle of the operation: How does it work? Where do you do it? Will others be able to see where the surgery was done? We'll cover those here.

Trabeculectomy means removing a piece of the trabecular meshwork. It follows a long line of similar operations done since 1900. Their general purpose is to let water leak from inside the eye, out through the wall of the eye and under the covering tissue (conjunctiva) where it slowly leaks into the tears. Peter Watson of England developed the concept of the present surgery in the 1960s and improvements have been added about every 5 years since then. To summarize what is done (Figure 23), the eye has two layers near the junction of the white and colored part: these are the conjunctiva, a flexible tissue a lot like sandwich wrap, and the sclera, the strong white part of the eye. The surgeon cuts and folds back the conjunctiva, makes an apron-shaped flap half-way down within the sclera, folds the flap back and removes tissue enough to make a hole into the front chamber of the eye. The iris would plug up this hole from the inside, so a piece of iris is removed right under the hole. The flap is put back and sewn in place with tiny nylon sutures that act to keep all the aqueous from running out immediately—this is essentially an adjustable valve. Then, the conjunctiva is sewn back in place to cover the area and to begin sopping up the fluid coming out, like a sponge.

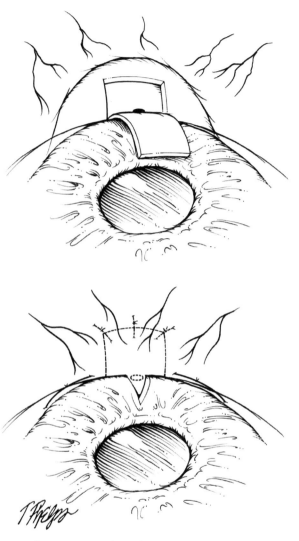

Figure 23: Drawing illustrating trabeculectomy surgery. Upper drawing shows the conjunctiva is folded back and a flap is made in the sclera, part-way through. A hole is made into the eye (small dark oval under flap) and a piece of the iris is removed. In the lower drawing, the flap in the sclera and the conjunctiva are sewn back in place. The hole under the flap is shown as a dotted oval. 3 sutures are shown holding the sclera flap. These can be loosened after surgery to adjust the eye pressure.

The area of trabeculectomy is always under the upper eyelid – there's room up there for 2 of them if the first one doesn't work long enough. Most often others can't see where it was done, since it's covered by the eyelid. It can be an area that is elevated some by the fluid coming out and it usually has fewer blood vessels than the surrounding conjunctiva, so it looks whiter there. Eye surgeons call this the bleb, since it looks something like a bubble (Figure 24). We tell patients it will be there, but often they forget and six months later they are startled to raise their eyelid and notice the bleb. My wife calls this the Saturday Morning I Just Noticed My Bleb Emergency Call. It's always good to be able to reassure someone that we call the bleb a success, not a problem.

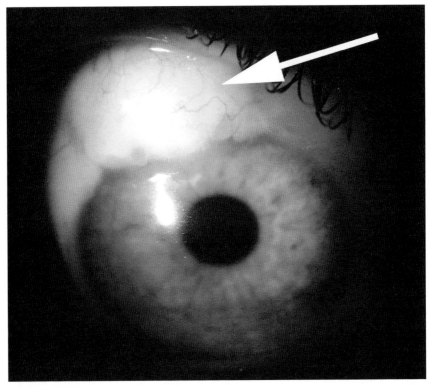

Figure 24: Photograph of the area of trabeculectomy glaucoma surgery called the bleb (arrow). This is where fluid from inside the eye slowly comes out to keep the eye pressure lower. Most blebs are smaller than this example, which is shown so that the bleb can be more easily appreciated in a picture.

The trabeculectomy works when more aqueous fluid gets out of the eye and the new pressure is at or below the target (see **What is the target pressure?**). This means we have to fool the body into thinking it healed the opening shut when it didn't. Several things help to do this. One is how the flap is constructed. Another is that the eye's own aqueous fluid actually prevents healing, for the same reason that the iris doesn't heal shut iridotomy made with the laser. Third, we often put a strong anti-healing medicine on the eye at the time of surgery to discourage the internal opening from closing—this is the drug mitomycin-C. Finally, you will be putting anti-inflammation eye drops on every 2 hours for a couple weeks and then slowly decreasing it, which is the final and important step in making the operation work by keeping the hole open.

Early after surgery, we want the pressure to stay a bit over the target. It helps to fool the eye into thinking nothing happened. So on the one day, one week, and three week visits (there are about four visits all together), you may hear that the pressure is still higher than the target. We plan that, and lower it into the target range gradually. Remember that the flap of sclera was sewn with stitches—these can be released or melted to reduce their tension, so aqueous flows faster through the hole and the pressure falls. Some surgeons use releasable sutures that are removed during a standard eye exam without any pain. My favorite is to melt them under the surface with a tiny laser delivery, one at a time.

We can tell a lot about how the operation is working during the first weeks, but I like to say that I'll be able to tell you that we have a success in five years. By six to eight weeks, you'll be stopping all eye drops to see if the target is achieved. I have patients whose trabeculectomy is still working 30 years later, so we're in this for the long haul. Unfortunately, they all don't work for three decades. About 20% of trabeculectomies fail to control pressure by one year. After that, about one in 25 (4%) stops working each year. In a review of trabeculectomies done at the Wilmer Glaucoma Center of Excellence, with lots of different patients, some with very difficult problems, nearly two-thirds were still at their target and on no medicine four to five years afterwards, and no further surgery had been needed for the eye.

The main issues that come up after trabeculectomy (other than pressure failure) are: too low a pressure (sometimes due to a leaking bleb), early or later infection, discomfort caused by the bleb area, and bleeding inside the eye. Low pressure can cause blurred or variable vision, and this can happen both with a large hole in the bleb wall or without it. When pressure is very low, the layers of the eye wall can fail to stay in their normal position plastered together. They drift off into the eye, causing dark shadows that block vision. These are called choroidal detachments and they do not harm the eye permanently. Another condition can occur when the pressure is low called hypotony maculopathy. In this, the back of the eye becomes slightly folded (like a balloon losing air), blurring vision. While these are uncommon events, they sometimes can lead to permanent changes in vision. Low pressure (hypotony) is fixed by removing the conjunctiva over the bleb, advancing the conjunctiva to cover the area, and restitching the flap back tightly. This is most often successful and in the vast majority, vision is improved and the target pressure is still achieved. Any operation can have bacteria enter the eye during surgery. These are most often the patient's own bacteria that normally live on the eye's surface. We take lots of steps to keep them out of the eye and to sterilize the eye surface just prior to surgery, but one in 1,000 or so operations have an infection develop in the first month. We let patients know the signs of infection that they should look for. When they call us promptly about such symptoms, we are very successful at treating infection without bad results. In an infection, the eye has pain, a big increase in redness, a sticky discharge on the lids (pus), and vision often is much worse. Any two or three of these should lead to a fast phone call to the doctor, even on Saturday night.

Late infection can happen with trabeculectomy and to a lesser extent with tube-shunt surgery even months to years after surgery. Why this is true makes sense if you visualize the operation: it's a new channel through the eye wall from the inside chamber, then under the flap, and finally under the conjunctiva. If bacteria can get through the first layer of conjunctiva, they can swim or drift inside the eye much easier than in a normal eye where the white sclera is intact. It's obviously still hard for bacteria to get in, because among thousands of trabeculectomies, there are few infections. The rate is about one in one thousand operations each year after surgery. Again, one key to minimizing the risk of infection is to have patients recognize symptoms of infection and call in quickly. A bleb with an overt leak in the conjunctiva makes infection even easier--it's a free ride into the eye from bacteria living around the eyelids and tears.

For about a year after any surgery on any body part, the nerves in the area have to regrow and during that time things feel different. Most often this is minor and can be soothed by taking artificial tear drops (over the counter type). Many patients describe this as "it doesn't quite feel like my old eye yet". It is very uncommon for us to have to do surgery to fix these feelings, although occasionally the bleb gets too high or extends too far down all around the white of the eye and needs to be revised.

There are those for whom trabeculectomy works better and those in whom it's unlikely to win. The success rate is higher in eyes without past surgery and in older persons. It's like a senior discount: older persons heal worse, so the surgery works better. It's not so favorable if you scar a lot, have had other past eye surgery, or have ongoing inflammation in the eye or some form of secondary glaucoma. For reasons that aren't fully understood, African-derived persons do worse (see **Special section for African-derived persons**).

Cataract and trabeculectomy

The good news is that cataract surgery is really successful at removing a hazy lens from your eye, replacing it with a new artificial lens, and getting your vision back to its best possible. The bad news is that glaucoma patients can get more cataract sooner in life than those without glaucoma. Part of this is just the disease, and part is due to the treatments speeding up cataract. Cataract happens faster whether you are treated with drops or with surgery. Remember: if you don't stop glaucoma damage, you will lose vision you cannot get back. Cataract vision loss is reversible.

157

When patients who have had trabeculectomy are studied, they develop a need for cataract surgery in the next five years frequently. So, if there is already cataract there in an eye that is in need of trabeculectomy, we can do the two operations rolled into one. The end result success rate for the combined operation is about the same as for persons who had trabeculectomy alone, later got cataract, then had the second operation to remove cataract. And, combining them together means only one operation, not two. But, doing them together adds complexity and a few more potential problems, so you don't want to take out the lens (cataract) unless you've considered the options with the surgery.

There is some evidence that removing cataract by surgery actually lowers eye pressure a bit. Not as much as having a full additional trabeculectomy, however. So, if you need a substantially lower target pressure and you have a removable cataract, the cataract operation alone will not always do the trick. Of course, if you can avoid the combination trabeculectomy, you avoid the risks of trabeculectomy, like too low pressure and late infection. You will want to consider this carefully with the surgeon before deciding.

Tube-Shunt Surgery

Tube-shunt surgery does the same thing as trabeculectomy: it lets aqueous humor out of the eye. It was designed to work when the normal area where fluid would drain out in a trabeculectomy has been scarred by prior surgery. The device that is implanted is a tiny tube of flexible plastic that goes into the front chamber of the eye and leads back to a flat area of plastic that is sewn to the sclera of the eye far back behind (Figure 25). Fluid drains out of the eye, into the tube (Figure 26) and is sopped up in a large cavity that forms around the flat plastic plate back behind the eye. Some brands of tube-shunts have a valve inside the tube that is intended to keep the pressure from going too low soon after surgery, while with others the surgeon blocks the tube off with a temporary stitch that dissolves about four to six weeks after surgery.

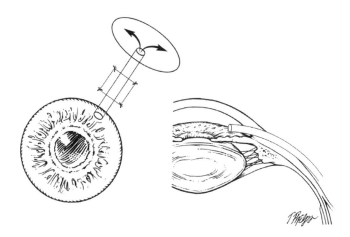

Figure 25: Drawings of tube—shunt operation seen from the front (left) and from a cutaway view (right). A tube is placed into the front chamber of the eye, leading back behind the eye where a reservoir is created to drain off fluid and lower eye pressure.

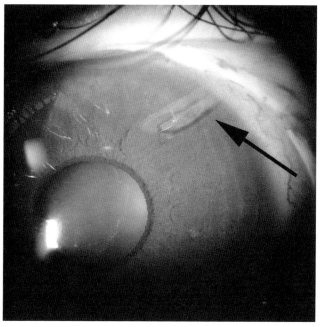

Figure 26: Photograph of a tube shunt (arrow) as seen inside the eye in front of the brown iris.

Materials that are sewn onto the eye tend to work their way out, that is, they can erode free to the surface, so the tube portion is covered by material from donated eye bank eyes that has been sterilized. The conjunctiva covers over the procedure and most often no sutures need removal.

Most of the pre- and post-operative experiences for trabeculectomy and tube-shunt surgery are similar. A recent study randomly compared tube-shunt surgery to trabeculectomy in eyes that had undergone prior surgery of some kind. In those eyes, the tube cases did as well or better than trabeculectomy in a number of areas, though each kept the pressure at or below target at about the same rate. The tube cases had fewer eyes that went too low in pressure, while the trabeculectomies needed fewer glaucoma eye drops in the short to medium term. Infections would be expected more often with trabeculectomy, but tube operations still can have the tube erode to the surface and may need recovering or removal. As many as one in ten eyes with tube—shunts have double vision for a time. This is because the materials sewn on prevent the eyes from moving together.

Presently, studies are ongoing to see if tube-shunt operations might be good for eyes that have not had prior surgery. In some eyes, trabeculectomy might be a poor first choice—for example, eyes with bad inflammation, eyes with secondary glaucoma that have new blood vessels growing, and some eyes of children with glaucoma (see **Secondary glaucoma** and **Children and glaucoma**).

Diode laser ciliodestruction

Laser treatment can decrease the amount of aqueous humor that is being formed by the ciliary body. The laser is delivered only in the operating room, due to the pain that would be caused. The laser can be delivered from the outside of the eye by passing through the surface of the eye along a fiber optic cable and focused inside the eye by a special probe (Figure 27). Or, the laser can be delivered by a probe that is inserted into the front or the mid-portion of the eye with the viewing done either through the pupil or by an endoscope making a picture on a TV screen. In all 3 situations, the laser burns the tissue of the ciliary body and decreases how much fluid is being made. We treat about 2/3 of the area making fluid so that all fluid production doesn't stop. In that case, the eye would have too low a pressure.

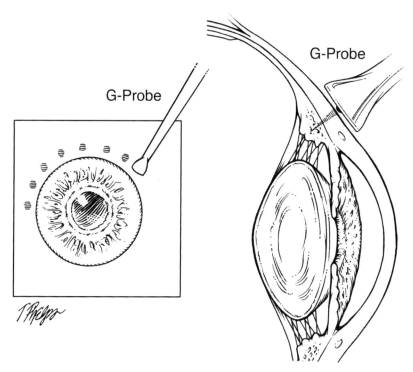

Figure 27: Drawings of laser ciliodestruction performed from outside the eye in front view (left) and cutaway view (right). The laser energy comes down the G-probe and is focused on the ciliary body inside the eye, in a series of applications in a circle around the eye (shaded circles in left drawing). The energy is focused on the ciliary body (right drawing), where aqueous humor is produced, lowering pressure.

The treatment, especially the one done from the outside of the eye, is quick (about 10 minutes), but it is most often reserved for those glaucoma eyes in which neither trabeculectomy nor tube—shunting would work well. This is because the treatment causes damage inside the eye, releasing parts of the destroyed tissues into the central cavity of the eye where they cause inflammation and debris that must settle down and be engulfed before vision is back to what it was before surgery. Furthermore, eyes that have had this treatment sometimes develop swelling in the central vision area, the macula, and reading vision is affected badly. Rarely the laser can lead to a very low eye pressure that can stay that way permanently.

But, when pressure lowering is needed and other treatments haven't worked, laser ciliary body treatment can save vision. It achieves the target pressure in two of three operations. When the target is not achieved, a repeat laser treatment can be done, treating more of the fluid-producing area. Sometimes there is a little more pain after this treatment than the other glaucoma surgeries, and sometimes the patient needs to use strong pain pills.

New procedures

There are a variety of newly proposed procedures to treat glaucoma, most of them involving ways to improve outflow of aqueous by treating the meshwork. There is a technique called the Trabectome that can improve aqueous outflow and lower pressure by removing a thin layer of trabecular tissue. A second new treatment called Canaloplasty widens the final canal at the end of the meshwork. A third new procedure called iStent puts a tiny tube inside the eye into the trabecular meshwork to improve its flow. Finally, there are some operations that are "almost trabeculectomy" but don't actually make a hole all the way inside the eye (viscocanalostomy, non-penetrating sclerectomy). None of these procedures is so much better than trabeculectomy that they have become the procedure of choice, though each has some positive aspects.

Can the treatments be worse than the disease?

TAKE HOME POINTS:

- **Some open angle glaucoma suspects should be followed closely without treatment**
- **You can always change treatments if one isn't right for you**
- **Pills marked with a "glaucoma caution" can usually be used—if the eye doctor checks them**
- **Steroids are especially dangerous for glaucoma patients, requiring monitoring pressure**

Eye treatments that can be stopped

A primary rule of medicine is "First, do no harm". We must continuously be thinking about whether things that are recommended as treatments are, on balance, better than doing nothing. My resident doctors in training like to joke that I take as many patients off eye drops as I put on them. By this, they mean that I often will try a unilateral stop trial (stopping the drops in one eye), just to see if they are really doing enough for the patient. You don't want to take things every day that aren't helping.

In recent research into who actually benefits from glaucoma treatment, my colleague at the Wilmer Glaucoma Center, Michael

Boland, makes the strong case that many persons over age 70 who are open angle glaucoma suspects could often be followed without eye drops—and lose no significant vision during the rest of their lives. So, it is not true as patients sometimes tell me: "once I start the eye drops I guess I'll always have to use them, right?" No, you can try them and if they're not right for you, you can stop, under certain conditions.

General body treatments that can affect glaucoma

There are hundreds of pills for which the FDA statements about the drug include a glaucoma caution, that is, they say that it may be dangerous for glaucoma patients to take them. Among these are the many medicines used for anxiety and psychological disorders, things like the serotonin reuptake inhibitors, the first of which was Prozac (fluoxetine). Apparently, there were reported examples of angle closure glaucoma that happened in those taking this pill. The same could occur with all the frequently used drugs that help with urinary incontinence and with some of the upper respiratory cold pills. For all of these, the risk is that the pupil might be dilated, and angle closure might result. But, for all those with open angles, these medications are perfectly fine. And, they're fine for any angle closure person who has already had an iridotomy (see **Acute angle closure crisis**).

So, what should you and your medical doctor do when you want to use a medication, but it has a glaucoma caution on the label? Call your ophthalmologist. In nearly every case, it will be fine to start the pill. The best approach is often to start it and have an eye exam in the next month to check on potential bad effects. If you know you have open angle glaucoma, you can take most medications that have a warning about glaucoma, but you need to be monitored if you start taking some of them.

Most worrisome for glaucoma patients or those at risk for glaucoma, are medications that deliver corticosteroid ("steroid") to your body. We use steroids as ways to treat a huge number of disorders, including arthritis, asthma, sinus trouble, and more serious general body disorders. Cortisone (prednisone) as a pill at full dosage can in fact cause eye troubles, but if they help your general condition, we can manage the effects. The eye issue closest to this discussion is an increase in eye pressure caused by steroids. This occurs in the more sensitive person even from nasal sprays and inhalers that have steroids. I have not seen it from injections into joints, but pills and particularly injections of steroid into the eye for various diseases will often increase eye pressure. The right answer is always to get the doctors talking to each other and watch things carefully.

There are more and more suggestions that how we control the blood pressure of persons can be relevant to open angle glaucoma. High blood pressure can kill you, so get it treated. But, we run across persons taking three or even four pill types for hypertension. One has to wonder if this is the same issue as we find with glaucoma drugs. If you forgot to take your pills when you saw the doctor, he/she might have added another one. If the same thing happened again, pretty soon you were being prescribed three or four of them. This happened to an older family relative of mine. She was found in her bathroom in the middle of the night, having fallen and hit her head on the sink. Turns out she was taking several pills for blood pressure (and one for sleep) and had just re-filled them after not having them all recently. Suddenly, a huge drop in blood pressure happened from taking everything (and the sleeping pill) and she wound up in the hospital. My point is that we should be using the right amount of medicine and taking it regularly, so that the doctor can tell how to give neither too much nor too little. It's as bad for a glaucoma patient to have a low blood pressure as to have high blood pressure (maybe worse). Lesson one, take your pills. Lesson two, don't get put on four medications when one or two will do the job if only you were taking them properly.

Are there treatments other than lowering eye pressure?

TAKE HOME POINTS:

- **Neuroprotection treatments will come in the future, but none is ready now**
- **Drugs and laser used in secondary glaucoma**
- **"Non-traditional" treatments: what you don't know can hurt you**

We are sometimes confronted with a patient who has obeyed all the rules of treatment, taking drops religiously, coming for exams on time, and still vision seems to be slowly declining. From large studies, we know that lowering the eye pressure significantly slows the progress of glaucoma so that most patients don't end up impaired. However, there is a limit to what lowering eye pressure can do. For one thing, in some persons when we lower it too much surgically, vision gets so blurred we have to operate to raise it back again.

It would be very important to develop treatments that add to pressure lowering, that protect ganglion cells from dying by making them less sensitive to the bad influences of glaucoma. I and many of my very bright colleagues have spent the last 38 years working on that problem. It is one of the highest priorities of the National Eye Institute and each of the non-governmental organizations that fund research into glaucoma. The word that is used for this kind of non-pressure lowering treatment is neuroprotection, meaning protecting the nerves in the eye.

The steps that have been taken so far involve several lines of work. First, we study how glaucoma affects human eyes, what seems to make it better or worse, and look for clues that can be studied in controlled laboratory research. Then, we develop models of glaucoma in individual cells in culture dishes, in pieces of the eye studied in the lab, and in animal models in animals that are as close to human glaucoma as possible. In each of these, we look for pathways that lead from some starting bad thing that glaucoma does, and step by step cause ganglion cells to die. We have found pathways that lead to ganglion cell death. There are also survival pathways that are activated when the injury starts and whose job it is keep the nerve cells alive. Your glaucoma could be helped either by blocking the death pathways or by strengthening the survival pathways.

I'll illustrate how far we've come along one pathway to point out an approach that could be tried in human glaucoma patients quite soon. It's fair to say that this is the best-studied potential new treatment, but I could list another 12 that have shown benefit all the way up to blocking glaucoma nerve cell death in animal models. In the section **How did you get glaucoma?**, we mentioned that the ganglion cell fiber is damaged in glaucoma as it passes out of the eye through the optic nerve head. When the fiber is injured there, its ability to carry messages from outside the eye back to the ganglion cell in the eye is blocked (obstructed axonal transport). The cell depends on receiving these messages every day to tell it what it going on up at the other end of its long fiber and to reassure it that it's connected to the right target cells in the brain.

When the messages don't arrive properly at the cell body, it triggers a response left over from life in the womb. When you were a fetus, fibers knew that they had gone to the right target cell in the brain by receiving the right messages or neurotrophic factors (called names like BDNF and CNTF). Baby nerve cells that didn't receive the BDNF message thought that they were connected incorrectly, and evolution developed a mechanism for getting rid of these mistargeted nerve cells. They committed suicide by a genetic program in their DNA. This cell suicide process is called apoptosis. It sounds horrifying but it is actually an important tool our bodies use to keep only healthy cells and to develop correctly. In glaucoma, when the message is blocked and BDNF levels fall in the cell body, this program is activated and the cell commits apoptosis. We found this pathway was active in both animals and humans with glaucoma. The logical solution would be to provide more BDNF, which we did by inserting the gene for it into the retina of rats. Presto! Fewer ganglion cells died in those rats with lots of BDNF. A similar experiment worked with the factor called CNTF. The reason that's important is that a company has developed a way to give CNTF continuously to the eye and is already treating humans who have retinitis pigmentosa with it so see if it helps. Their ingenious system is a little capsule that can be sewn inside the eye. This is not trivial, but certainly possible for many eyes without interfering with vision. Inside the capsule are human cells that are engineered to constantly produce CNTF. The recipient eye's defense mechanism can't kill these cells by immune rejection, because they are inside the capsule, but the CNTF gets out to bathe the retina. Such capsules have been safely put in human eyes for a year or more without ill effects.

This is only one of a number of ways that an implanted device, or a drug taken as a pill, or a viral carrier containing a new gene could be used to attempt neuroprotection in glaucoma. There has already been one trial of 1,000 patients with a pill that might have worked. Unfortunately, it didn't work with the drug called Memantine. We and other researchers are working very hard with some drug companies to try other approaches that could work. For example, the same viral carrier particle that put the CNTF into rats in our lab experiments has been used to put another gene into the eyes of human patients with a disease called Leber's congenital amaurosis, with great benefit to their vision. This is called gene therapy, and some form of it will surely be used in the future. With the millions of glaucoma patients, there should be plenty of reason for drug companies to help us to develop new treatments.

The problem is that we are impatient (and I'm at least as impatient as all my patients are) for a breakthrough in neuroprotection. This leads, however, to behavior that doesn't make sense. For example, well before we found out that Memantine, the failed neuroprotection drug, didn't work, lots of eye doctors decided to start prescribing it for their patients. This was possible because the drug was FDA approved to treat dementia, so it is legal to write prescriptions in what is called off-label use. This means that using it for glaucoma is not approved by the FDA, because there is no evidence it will help. This kind of prescribing is legal and is frequently done, as long as the patient knows that the drug hasn't been shown to help their problem. My opinion, however, is that if we don't know it will help, how do we know it won't hurt? Giving someone a drug without knowing the side effects on their eye and on their glaucoma is taking a risk without proven benefit.

But, at least using Memantine off label is using a drug that we know what is in each pill and whose general body bad effects have been studied scientifically. Use of other nutriceuticals, herbal remedies, and alternative treatments is another realm altogether. There is not a single one of the so-called treatments in these areas that has ever been shown scientifically to benefit glaucoma. Vitamins were shown not to help anything about glaucoma in a large, controlled research study. And, when you buy such a product, neither you nor I have any idea what is in it. I have heard from patients taking Ginko biloba, Echinacea, St Johns' Wort, and fish oil that they do it because they are "natural products, and after all, it can't hurt, can they?" Companies or web sites that sell these products have no extermal regulation system for what is in the product. Many of you read about the addition of melamine, a plastic component and poison of the kidneys, to milk products in China, killing many children. We have regulations on things that we take as medicine for a reason. Someone could cut their lawn today, put the clippings in a capsule and sell it to you at a health store or web site as an herbal medicine. I once had a patient tell me that he was taking a pill called "MK 801". I was intrigued, because I knew that a lab experiment in rats had shown benefit to rat glaucoma by dosing them with MK801 (the designation for a particular chemical in the same family as Memantine). Some enterprising Internet site was selling a white pill labeled as this chemical to gullible (and desperate) patients. The truth is that if the patient were actually taking MK801 in the dose it said, he would have died from it. MK801 is highly toxic, and the dose needed to help rats nearly killed them. Some of these herbals have bad effects that are unpredictable, like blocking the effects of birth control pills and causing strokes. It's not true that "it can't hurt".

One study of a series of "herbal" medicines that were analyzed scientifically found that some contained none of the supposed active ingredient, others contained much more than the stated amount. If you were taking insulin for diabetes, would you take 10 times more one day and none the next, without knowing which you were doing? The FDA web site lists a similar study, titled: "Tainted Products Marketed as Dietary Supplements" (http://www.fda.gov/downloads/ForConsumers/ConsumerUpdates/UCM236998.pdf)

One book written by a glaucoma patient for other glaucoma patients has actively advocated the benefit of holistic and alternative treatments. Anecdotal testimonials by individuals who claim to have been helped are not reasons to do something. If you wish to be a supporter of the development of truly acceptable new treatments for glaucoma, don't waste money on things that have no evidence to help you. Donate the money to a research group studying future neuroprotection for glaucoma in legitimate research laboratories.

One of the most frequently asked questions about unapproved treatments for glaucoma is whether marijuana really helps. After all, several states now permit use of "medical marijuana". The bottom line is that you don't want to smoke or swallow pot to treat your glaucoma. It is true that marijuana has some power to lower eye pressure. There are several good reasons why it's not useful. First, no one can standardize how much potency it has—the chemicals in pot are a very complex mixture of things called cannabinoids, and no one can figure out which single one of them alone might be approved as an official FDA drug. Second, you can't separate the pressure-lowering from being stoned, and you would have to be high all day, every day to get the effect on glaucoma. Third, if you smoke it, you ruin your lungs and increase your lung cancer risk. Fourth, you're at risk for ingesting whatever insecticide someone put on it. Finally, you'd be supporting some drug cartel in most cases.

How should I change my life?

> **TAKE HOME POINTS:**
>
> - **Don't smoke and limit sunlight exposure (even though they don't relate to glaucoma)**
> - **Do perform aerobic exercise**
> - **Do no exercises with your head below your heart**
> - **Breathe continuously through all exercise (don't hold your breath)**
> - **Special cautions for musical wind instrument players**
> - **Use your eyes all you want (Mom was wrong about this one)**

"You mean I'm going to have to take these drops for the rest of my life?" For those choosing eye drops, this is a major reality of how glaucoma will change your daily activities, though if it's one 5 minute period getting the drop in once per day, and the occasional refill of the bottle at drug store or prescription plan, that isn't a huge time commitment. More than anything, it is the knowledge that something (another thing) is wrong with our body that is depressing, at first. The more we realize that glaucoma can be managed and generally kept from changing our life, the less depressing it should be.

Often, I am asked: "What else can I do in my daily activities that will help my glaucoma?" In comparing glaucoma to other diseases, especially the major eye diseases, there are only a few things that you will wish to consider. We know, for example, that cigarette smoking and sunlight exposure are both big causes of the eye diseases called cataract and age-related macular degeneration. Interestingly, these are not related to glaucoma. You still shouldn't smoke and you shouldn't be outside without eye protection, because these diseases happen to people of your age, too. But, in extensive studies of personal habits, we and others have found that diet, alcohol consumption, and caffeine intake are pretty much unrelated to causing glaucoma or making it worse. Clearly, eating a healthy diet containing fruits and vegetables and limiting booze and caffeine to a small amount per day will help you to live longer and healthier. So do that for yourself and to last long enough to watch your grandkids grow up. If you drink more than one caffeinated beverage per day, knock it down to one and make the rest of what you drink caffeine-free.

One major thing you can do that is proven to lower eye pressure and improve blood flow to the brain and the eye is aerobic exercise. This means doing something at least four times per week for more than 20 minutes that raises your pulse rate to a level that makes your heart work. Generally, it means walking, swimming, biking, or stationery machining at a level that keep you a bit out of breath. You should be able to talk to the person with whom you're running or walking, but with difficulty. The term aerobic exercise was coined by Dr Kenneth Cooper and his Institute's web site, (http://www.cooper-aerobics.com) is a source of information on how you can figure out how to do the right thing for your heart and your retinal ganglion cells. First, check with your medical doctor before starting anything. Second, you may wish to be referred to a physical therapist for good hints on what and how to do it. Third, pick something that you really will do four times a week. If you hate to swim, don't try that. If you can't afford a health club membership, pick walking. Fourth, get a partner. When I ran marathons, one of my training systems was that I knew two guys were going to show up to run with me at my back door every dark, cold morning. If I thought that rolling over in bed and going back to sleep was a good idea, having them bang in the kitchen door reminded me to get my running shoes on. You will enjoy walking and talking with someone or a group more than solo. Fifth, make a standard time when the exercise is going to happen. With my busy schedule of job and kids, I had to simply get up 45 minutes earlier every day. In studies with older adults with early glaucoma, eye pressure fell by two points or so as they began consistent exercise. It's almost as good as adding another eye drop to protect your vision. Get off the couch!

Exercises which you should avoid are anything in which you are upside down or your head is below your heart during the exercise. For example, head stands or down-facing dog pose in Yoga cause your eye pressure to be twice or three times higher than normal. While there has been no study to show that yoga leads to worsening of glaucoma, there are plenty of other Yoga poses to decrease your stress level. In fact, our research group is now studying whether practicing yoga could lower eye pressure. Holding your breath while exerting yourself (called the Valsalva maneuver, like straining on the toilet) is also a time when your eye pressure goes sky high. So, if you lift weights for exercise, which is generally a good idea to maintain bone density, make it low weights with more repetitions of lifting, rather than heavy weights that make you grunt. A similar breath-holding problem applies to those playing the larger wind musical instruments like the French horn. One study suggested that there was a greater chance of glaucoma in symphonic wind players. If you play a brass instrument, it makes sense to have frequent checks of pressure, optic nerve head and visual field.

Your Mom may have told you not to read so much or you'd ruin your eyes. Mom was right about a lot of things and here she was only half right. Persons between the ages of eight and 15 develop more near-sightedness from close eye work if they have some inherent tendency to it. But, for the adult glaucoma patient, there is no reason to think that using the eyes is harmful. Read away. You can rot your brain by watching reality TV, but it won't hurt your glaucoma.

What does low vision treatment have to offer?

TAKE HOME POINTS:

- **Taking the step to meet with a Low Vision specialist takes willingness to change**
- **It's what's next after regular glasses don't help**
- **Reading can still be fun, but with changes in how it's done**
- **Safety in walking and living means keeping your independence**
- **Whether you still drive or not should be determined with expert advice**

Some years ago, my godmother, whose art projects had always graced her home, developed a severe vision problem in her 80s. Unable to read normal print with standard glasses, she felt that it might be no longer possible to lead a "normal" life. Fortunately, two things made it possible for her, now 97, to continue to send me lovely hand-written letters, to do her finances and to surf the Internet. First, she has the wonderful capability of adjusting to change. That isn't easy for all of us, as I realize with every passing year. Persons whose vision has changed forever for the worse, can easily fall into the trap of feeling sorry for themselves. People keep searching in vain for a cure and a way to make it like it always was.

I hear them just keep asking for "a different pair of glasses that will let me see normally." There are no magic glasses. My godmother was willing to try something new if it let her enjoy life more.

She fortunately had an eye doctor who recommended that she seek Low Vision consultation and she lives in a city that has a fine office for that. Many eye doctors try their medicines, their lasers and their surgery, and, when no further "treatment" will help, the patient hears the message: "there's nothing more I can do." That's hard for doctors to admit, since we spend our whole lives trying to help and (like everyone else) we're lousy losers. However, it is not the end of the line. After the initial shock wears off and acceptance begins, the next step is to seek low vision rehabilitation services.

No one wants to think of themselves as "low vision" or "blind", and the images of white canes, seeing-eye dogs, and dark glasses may even invoke our pity, but, surprisingly, our research has shown that 37% of people seeking low vision services nationally have only mild visual impairment and are simply not satisfied with their present visual function. Even a little vision problem can become frustrating when you just need to read the account number off a credit card. I find that many of my patients simply don't want to give vision rehabilitation a try. My argument is that they have little to lose and a lot to gain. You don't know what can be done to make your life better without finding out what's out there. Understanding what treatments, practical aids, technology and training that physicians, occupational therapists and orientation and mobility specialists have to offer, can be empowering. With that said, one visit to a low vision clinic will not undo the effects of vision loss from glaucoma nor will it cure you. Like any treatment, if you are told about things to do and you don't want to do them, you can walk away. In fact, a vast majority of my patients who have gone to our Wilmer Lions Vision Center for consultation tell me that there were beneficial treatments and suggestions that improved the quality of their lives. Like any form of rehabilitation, success may involve change, and that may be a lot to ask for. This is where the rubber meets the road. A positive attitude, an open mind and good support can make a world of difference during this process.

Problems reading, driving, and walking in dimly lit restaurants are common complaints. Low vision rehabilitation addresses each activity by using lenses, lighting, reverse telescopes, special filters, camera, cell phone technology, and adaptive strategies. Nowadays, there's a lot of equipment out there to improve visual function — magnifiers with LED lights, video magnification, software, etc. To assess rehabilitation potential and make treatment recommendations, specialists can be helpful in directing the approach before spending money on devices that are not right for you. Buying things off the Internet might sound simple, but you can't tell what you need and everyone wants to sell you their product. I wouldn't think of buying a new car without test-driving it first. Devices may not be the solution. Training on adaptive techniques and "low-tech" solutions may be what's necessary. You really don't need your vision for everything — someday we'll be able to drive without it. For now, however, instead of getting frustrated with getting the toothpaste on the toothbrush, just squeeze the paste on your finger first and then wipe it on the brush. A low vision specialist has only your best interests at heart and is the best person to direct this part of your care.

Before vision loss, you probably used reading glasses either as part of "bifocals" (now mostly progressively changing power lenses) or separate reading glasses. Glaucoma often leaves the ability to read individual letters or words pretty much intact, but constricts the usable area of reading vision to a tiny tube of good vision in the center. On occasion you may notice that you miss the beginning of words or it is harder to keep your place when going to the next line of print on the left. When my glaucoma colleague, Dr. Pradeep Ramulu, developed special tests for continuous reading, he found that glaucoma patients start out okay, but slow down much more than others their age by 15 minutes into their reading. This is exactly what we had heard from patients over many years: "I get really tired quickly when trying to read." This is where careful examination can make all the difference, as it may be dry eye or cataracts that are causing the problem, rather than the glaucoma. Fortunately, the ability to see small print is often retained, but it is the loss of contrast sensitivity, the sense that someone has taken some of the ink out of the printer that's annoying. You may find reading red writing on a blue background is impossible. This loss of contrast sensitivity is often the culprit in problems driving at night and recognizing faces at a distance.

Low vision specialists make things better through a variety of "work-arounds" and solutions, such as better ways to light the page you're reading, and moving the book to the optimal distance for what you're trying to see. Task lighting is often the most effective solution to enhance reading. Directed-source lights, like the full-spectrum and LED, positioned properly and close to the book, may dramatically improve reading ability. Some of our patients even contract with electricians to make lighting modifications in their home that can make all the difference. For the most part, people with glaucoma need a lot of light, but undirected light can be troublesome in certain situations.

Glaucoma patients are very bothered by glare, meaning light that comes into the eye from the side or the top, away from the center part you're trying to use to see. Indoor fluorescent lighting at superstores, driving in and out of shady areas or adjusting to changing light when walking out of a movie theater can be worrisome and even scary at times. Understanding the effects of changing light and preparing accordingly can be helpful. Glare outdoors is best handled by hats with a brim (baseball caps or a visor are great). Sunglasses that are too dark can be worse than not having them on. They cut down the light coming directly where you want to see, but let in light coming in from the side (the glare producing stuff). If you don't like hats to block glare, get wrap-around glasses where either the lenses or the frames block light coming from the sides. Each person is different, and the choice of filter color and light transmission can make a difference. Glare evaluations can be performed as part of low vision assessment.

If reading small print has gotten harder, magnification may be helpful and prescribed in the form of spectacles, hand-held devices and computer adaptations. For some with glaucoma, however, bigger print is not always better. If reading books and newspapers are important to you and magnification is not effective, than you may wish to attempt listening to Talking Books. They are read by wonderful actors and it is a great way to continue to enjoy the classics or the latest best sellers. Talking Books are widely available and many local libraries and many have converted from the traditional cassette tapes to providing very easy-to-operate digital players. The digital tapes of interest are sent to your home so there's no need to drive to the library. Because of computer use and the advent of Kindles and IPads, reading with vision impairment has been revolutionized. Best yet, when the eyes tire, turn on Text-to-Speech, sit back, relax, and listen. I always tell my patients, that there has never been a better time in history to live life with vision impairment.

The great thing about watching TV and using a computer is that you can make it easier with the right kind of lens correction and by changing the device. Often using glasses prescribed for the computer, changing your work distance, getting a bigger screen, or using the right kind of software that enhances the font or reads aloud will make it the activity less frustrating. Understanding what is effective for you can make life more fulfilling.

Judging stairs, steps, and curbs and walking safely can be challenging with vision loss from glaucoma. In studies that Dr. Ramulu and others working with us at Wilmer have done, we find that glaucoma patients who have significant loss of vision walk more slowly and, unfortunately, bump into things more often. People comment that they are more cautious when walking because they are afraid of falling. Orientation and mobility specialists, occupational therapists specializing in vision impairment and physical therapists can assist with fall prevention and balance, thus improving your mobility safety. Your doctor or therapist may recommend something as simple as removing the bifocal and prescribing distance-only glasses. You can be more confident while walking after low vision assistance by learning how to use your remaining vision, by scanning effectively within your limited view and by considering the use of a walking stick or cane when out at night or in unfamiliar places. Home safety is the key to avoiding a fall that breaks a hip and puts you in the hospital. You can have a therapist who visits your home and makes many helpful suggestions about how to live independently and as normally as possible with limited vision. Some of the logical things that we don't immediately think of, for example, are the removal of cords that trip us up or sliding rugs.

Driving is one of the most important abilities for many in our culture, allowing independent living in our present home setting. But how safe are you driving with whatever glaucoma has caused in your vision? Do you know what you don't see? Many people with visual loss modify their own driving by limiting themselves to driving in the daytime and or only in familiar areas. Even with these restrictions, critical errors may occur. In one study of seniors, our group found that a substantial number of glaucoma patients had given up driving entirely. For some of them, this was probably for the best, as they could not see well enough to drive safely. As older age is associated with slower reaction times and physical limitations, it may be a good choice to find other ways to travel and shop. However, some patients who we found had given up driving seemed to have vision and capability that otherwise should not have been limiting. Legal doesn't mean safe and safe doesn't mean legal when it comes to driving. Talk with your vision rehabilitation physician. There are facilities available for testing your ability to drive with your present vision that will show you and experts that you continue to qualify to drive safely (or not).

A very common thing that persons with significant vision loss from glaucoma and other eye problems have is seeing things that aren't there. As many as one third of those with major vision loss experience seeing patterns, shapes, objects, and even people that they know are not real. These are not a sign of dementia and are not hallucinations in the sense of having a mental problem. I'm always glad when a patient trusts me enough to mention this, as older people fear that if they tell their children what they are seeing that the family with think that they have "lost it". These images are quite simply the product of your brain not getting visual stimulation from big areas of the view of the world from which the brain was used to "hearing". The phenomenon is named after a French doctor, Charles Bonnet. Patients described seeing patterns like the shape of tiles in a floor, like leafless trees against a winter sky, or images of realistic objects. As opposed to actual hallucinations, where the person being seen might talk to you, these are all visual things. It's as if the part of your brain devoted to vision gets bored when it doesn't get enough input. So, it plays back patterns and "movies" of past experience into the blind zones. This happens most often when we are not thinking about much, and staying very engaged in other activities makes it happen less. However, there is no way to stop it, despite some suggestions that strong psychoactive drugs can decrease it. We tell patients that once you understand what it is, you can hopefully "enjoy the show" without worrying that you're losing touch.

Vision loss is scary and can lead to disability and depression in some cases. In our recent research, there is evidence of depressed mood in about 22-25% of people seeking vision rehabilitation services. Depression is more common among seniors overall, but having visual difficulties makes it more likely. Seeking psychological counseling and treatment is appropriate. Some of the frustration from vision loss can be decreased by seeking vision rehabilitation services and incorporating devices and adaptive strategies in to daily life. Just remember, people born totally blind have fulfilling lives. The difference in glaucoma is often one's ability to adapt, just like my godmother.

Children and glaucoma

TAKE HOME POINTS:

- **Glaucoma in children runs in families, but not with one specific pattern or gene**
- **Signs of glaucoma in babies are big eyes and cloudy looking corneas**
- **Kids with glaucoma have too much tearing and hate any bright lights**
- **Specific surgery is the first treatment for many children with glaucoma**

Glaucoma in children could take up an entire book all on its own (and there are some good professional texts). Here, I will only hit on the most important points. Children are affected by glaucoma in less than one in a thousand births. No one actually has good figures on it, but as with other forms of glaucoma, if there is another affected family member, particularly a relative who got glaucoma as a youngster, the chance is much greater. In one study we did, 10% of children with glaucoma had one or more affected young or old family member with glaucoma.

Second, to identify that glaucoma has happened to a child isn't easy, but there are some typical signs. Children's eyes get bigger when eye pressure is higher, so their whole eye looks big. Second, the clear front of the eye (cornea) gets cloudy when pressure is high, so the eye looks white and the colored iris is harder to see. Something about how glaucoma affects kids causes them to hate bright lights and, in addition, their eyes have much more tearing than normal.

To diagnose what's going on in a child, we are fortunate that there is now a good pressure measuring device that works on them without anesthesia, the ICare tonometer. We also do ophthalmoscopy to evaluate the optic nerve head. When there is definite glaucoma in a child, our approach is often to suggest surgery as the best, first choice, for two reasons. First, a particular form of surgery (trabeculotomy or goniotomy) has a pretty high success rate. Second, if we can make the eye safe with surgery, it avoids years of eye drops daily.

There are children who have general body diseases that also have glaucoma as part of the disease. One of the more common is inflammatory disease, such as juvenile rheumatoid arthritis. Here, the approach should be a coordinated one between the specialist in arthritis and the eye specialist.

Premature babies have a particularly hard time developing their eyes normally and frequently need treatments for the inside of the eyes (retinopathy of prematurity), as well as later in life developing an unusual form of angle closure glaucoma.

Secondary glaucoma

TAKE HOME POINTS:

- **Secondary glaucoma raises eye pressure due to some additional cause in the eye or body**
- **Neovascular glaucoma comes from new blood vessels, due to diabetes or blocked blood vessels**
- **Injuries can lead to a glaucoma that needs ongoing treatment**
- **Inflammatory diseases can cause a secondary glaucoma**

Throughout this guide, we have mostly talked about the primary glaucomas, those that happen largely because of inherited traits and things we don't fully understand. By and large, there's really nothing else wrong in the eye (or the body) other than glaucoma in primary glaucoma.

Secondary glaucoma happens because of something else. It can be a something in the eye or in the body that affects the eye. If we total up all those with glaucoma in the world, the secondary ones are still a fair number, maybe 10% of all glaucoma. They much more often affect one eye and not both eyes, unlike primary open angle or angle closure that affect both eyes. All secondary glaucomas share the feature that the eye pressure is above normal due to something that causes abnormal outflow of aqueous.

Some people think we should classify some of the more common subgroups of open angle glaucoma as separate and secondary. This includes pigment dispersion syndrome and exfoliation syndrome (see **How did you get glaucoma?**). In this guide, we considered these as primary.

Probably the most common secondary glaucoma in the developed world are those that come from having new blood vessels grow in the meshwork and block outflow of aqueous: the neovascular glaucomas. We now know that this usually happens when the retina does not have enough blood supply. This leads to production of a chemical called vascular endothelial growth factor (VEGF) that floats around the inside of the eye, making new vessels to get blood flowing. The problem is that the new vessels grow the wrong places, messing up vision, detaching the retina and causing glaucoma. Diabetic persons sometimes have this happen. So do those persons who have a blockage in a main artery or vein in the eye (central retinal artery or vein occlusion). It also happens when the main neck artery to the brain blocks off (carotid artery occlusion). Nothing works to win against neovascular glaucoma unless we improve blood flow (open the carotid artery), decrease the need for blood in the retina (by lasering the retina), or inhibit VEGF (with injections of special blockers into the eye: Lucentis and Avastin). Once these things are done, we can treat this form of glaucoma with eye drops or with surgery and limit the damage.

Injuries to the eye are a frequent cause of both short-term glaucoma, due to ill effects of the injury, and long-term effects of damage to the meshwork by the blow. Frequent things that do this are bungee cord whip-backs into the eye, champagne corks for unwary celebrants, smaller athletic ball hits (squash, handball, lacrosse) for those who don't wear eye protection, and pellet and BB guns. All cause rips in the meshwork that scar it shut and make the pressure higher. Other associated injuries to the eye complicate the overall picture. Surgery is often needed to stop damage. Wearing safety glasses whenever you are involved in activities that can lead to eye injuries is a smart and safe way to avoid this.

Those with inflammation in the eye (uveitis) develop high eye pressure when inflammation or the treatments for inflammation (steroids) raise eye pressure. To make things more complex, inflammation sometimes also lowers eye pressure, so it can flip from high to low in an unpredictable way. Many inflammatory diseases can lead to glaucoma, including juvenile rheumatoid arthritis, sarcoidosis and other similar disorders. Medical and surgical glaucoma treatments are used, but are often more difficult to implement.

The list of secondary glaucomas is very long. One that has been of great interest to our group is the iridocorneal endothelial syndrome (ICE syndrome). Partly, it's a favorite because we gave it its name, and we have seen many persons with it over the years, even though it is not that common. It happens only in one eye, it looks somewhat like angle closure, and pressure can go quite high early in life, even in the 20s and 30s. The chief defect is an overgrowth of the cells on the back of the cornea (corneal endothelium) that blocks up outflow of aqueous. We treat with eye drops and often with surgery, sometimes having to replace the cornea with a transplant from an eye bank donor.

Special section for African-derived persons

TAKE HOME POINTS:

- **Open angle glaucoma is worse in African-derived persons**
- **Eye drops and surgery don't work quite as well in your eyes**
- **Medical care for glaucoma needs to do the job better**

Persons of color, those whose ancestors came from Africa, have a number of important issues that relate to glaucoma. Most importantly, you have three to four times more chance of having open angle glaucoma than other ethnicities, and it develops in your eyes at an earlier age than in others. Second, it is a more aggressive form of glaucoma, leading to vision loss and blindness more often. Third, there are some reasons to believe that even if you take your eye drops as others do that you won't quite get as much pressure lowering from the same dose. It seems that having more pigment in the eye soaks up the drugs that much more so they work less well. But, they do still work! Finally, many studies show that when we do glaucoma surgery (trabeculectomy), it works less often in African-derived persons.

So, given all the bad news, what else do we know and how can be overcome this? Well, one approach would be to give up and say that there's not much one can do and we should just kind of ignore the problem and hope it doesn't get us. That's a pretty human thing to do, but, it's a losing strategy. The answer to having higher rates of prostate and breast cancer is NOT to avoid having PSA blood tests and mammograms. The right answer is to follow the program. And eye doctors need help from you, because it seems, at least at the present time, that we don't know best how to get the message across to our African-derived patients.

We recently did studies on how patients take their drops for glaucoma and were surprised that our African-derived patients took them less frequently. This would be understandable, since on average African-derived persons have lower incomes, less health insurance, and less access to eye specialists. But, our studies were in persons who were educated, insured, and who got their eye drops for free as part of the study. And yet, when we clocked how well the drops got in, they did worse than other ethnicities. Not only that, but when we tried methods that would remind people to take their drops better, some improved a lot and others not so much. For African-derived patients, in general, the reminders we tried didn't work as well. This was even true when the doctor was an African-American woman.

This leads us to think that we aren't as culturally competent at communicating with our patients in ways that help them to prevent vision loss as well as we'd like. Attitudes toward disease must differ a lot among people. The medical community needs help in understanding what might work better than what we're doing now. I hope that those reading this will make suggestions that can improve our care of glaucoma.

Who should care for your glaucoma?

TAKE HOME POINTS:

- **Opticians make eyeglasses and fit frames**
- **Optometrists take care of glasses and medical eye problems, but do no laser procedures or surgery**
- **Ophthalmologists are medical doctors (M.D.) who study eight years after college and do surgery**
- **Board-certified ophthalmologists have passed rigorous tests on eye disease and surgery**
- **Members of the American Glaucoma Society did one or more years of special glaucoma education and are recognized experts**
- **Academic glaucoma specialists teach, do research, and only care for glaucoma patients**

Polls show that Americans have trouble telling the difference between the various kinds of eye care people. Let's make it easy. There is an optician, who makes glasses and frames, but doesn't look into the eye or treat eye disease. They essentially follow written instructions from eye doctors, and often perform important services in making glasses effective and comfortable. The optometrist goes to school for four years in studying normal eye function and eye diseases. They are not doctors of medicine (M.D.) and do not go to medical school to study general body disease. During their 4 year study, they typically get to examine people with eye disease under a faculty of other optometrists, but only in some optometric schools that partner with eye surgeons do they see persons who are being actively treated surgically. Many optometrists then take an extra year or more of specialized training in care of eye diseases. During the 1990s, state legislatures all over the U.S.A. passed laws permitting optometrists to prescribe eye drops for glaucoma, but not to treat glaucoma with laser or surgery. Only a small proportion of the prescriptions written for glaucoma in the U.S.A. are now written by optometrists alone. At the Wilmer Glaucoma Center, we have several excellent optometrist faculty members and work in a team approach, but the care of those with glaucoma is performed by ophthalmologists.

An ophthalmologist is an M.D. who went to four years of college, four years of medical school, one year of internship, then three years of specialized resident training in eye disease and eye surgery. After this training, an extensive written and oral set of examinations is given by the American Board of Ophthalmology, and only those who pass both are Board-certified ophthalmologists. You can find out if the ophthalmologist you want to see is Board-certified by going to the following web site (http://www.abms.org). You will need to provide an email address and a password that you make up to log in. The web site does not indicate which specialty board the doctor is certified, but if you are looking up an ophthalmologist, it is likely that it indicates Board certification in eye medicine.

Many ophthalmologists do one to three more years of specialized fellowship training in an area of eye disease, such as glaucoma care. This involves working in an office that has a large proportion of patients with glaucoma and observing and participating in laser and surgery procedures. Those fellowship-trained glaucoma specialists who are known to their colleagues as having excellent training and experience can be voted into membership in the American Glaucoma Society. At its web site (http://www.americanglaucomasociety.net/), there is a patient resource center that allows anyone to find the names and addresses of Glaucoma Society members. All board-certified ophthalmologists have studied and passed testing on all aspects of glaucoma care, and much of the care given to glaucoma patients in the U.S.A. is carried out by non-glaucoma specialists, including laser and surgical procedures. Some glaucoma specialists are full-time employees of Universities and teach fellows, residents, medical students and other eye doctors about glaucoma. Our Wilmer Institute Glaucoma Center of Excellence currently has seven full-time faculty members who only care for glaucoma and its associated problems. Most often, academic University glaucoma doctors see only persons with glaucoma and work with other advanced specialists at their Institution in other areas of ophthalmology. University faculty glaucoma specialists also perform research both with human patients and in laboratories.

Acknowledgements

I am grateful to my Glaucoma Center of Excellence colleagues and my family who made many helpful editorial comments for this guide, including Henry Jampel, Don Zack, David Friedman, Pradeep Ramulu, Michael Boland, Judith Goldstein, and David Quigley. Thanks to Elizabeth Bower for the cover photograph of the Wilmer Institute Smith Building and to Timothy Phelps of Art as Applied to Medicine, Johns Hopkins School of Medicine for the drawings.

Important Internet Links

For those who read this book and are motivated to make a contribution to "Wilmer Glaucoma Research", they can do so online at http://www.hopkinsmedicine.org/wilmer/charitable_giving/. At the section in the form "please designate my gift to" click on the "please select" and under the choices, click on "Glaucoma".

For those who wish to make an appointment for consultation about glaucoma with the Wilmer Glaucoma Center of Excellence doctors, the internet address is: http://www.hopkinsmedicine.org/wilmer/appointments/index.html. From that site, appointments can be made online or by telephone.

Dr Quigley accepts email questions about glaucoma at hquigley@jhmi.edu.

By late 2011, there will be an online version of this guide, with links to videos showing a variety of demonstrations, such as examination techniques, how to put in eye drops, and movies of glaucoma surgery. This can be viewed at no charge by going to the Glaucoma Service web page http://www.hopkinsmedicine.org/wilmer/

services/glaucoma.html and clicking on the link for <u>Glaucoma: What Every Patient Should Know</u>.

Other sites with authoritative information on glaucoma include:

http://www.nei.nih.gov   this is the site of the National Eye Institute, National Institutes of Health

http://www.glaucoma.org this is the site of a national charitable group serving glaucoma patients

http://www.ahaf.org/glaucoma/about/ this is the site of another charitable group serving glaucoma

Glossary

A

acetazolamide (Diamox): A medicine that lowers eye pressure in pill form, a carbonic anhydrase inhibitor.

acute angle closure crisis (attack): A sudden increase in eye pressure caused by several defects in movement of aqueous fluid in the eye. Symptoms are pain, redness, blurred vision and abnormal shaped pupil. A true emergency for which immediate care should be given.

adherence: The actual use of medicine by the patient.

aerobic exercise: Physical activity that raises the pulse rate substantially for a sustained period, which is known to lower eye pressure.

age-related macular degeneration (AMD): A disease affecting the center part of the vision by altering the nerve tissue called the retina and the underlying retinal pigment epithelium.

alpha adrenergic agonist eye drops: These eye drops reduce intraocular pressure by decreasing the production of aqueous humor and increasing its drainage through the uveoscleral pathway. Examples are brimonidine (Alphagan), apraclonidine (Iopidine), and dipivefrin (Propine).

angle: The junction of the iris and the cornea on the inside front part of the eye where aqueous fluid drains back into the blood stream from the eye along an area shaped like a circle.

angle closure: A mechanism that can lead to primary glaucoma in which the iris closes off the angle by moving forward.

angle closure glaucoma: A type of glaucoma caused by a blockade of movement of aqueous humor out of the eye as the iris is pushed against the trabecular meshwork.

anterior chamber: The front chamber of the eye between the cornea and iris that is filled with a liquid called aqueous humor.

anterior segment optical coherence tomography (ASOCT): An imaging method that shows the dynamic behavior of structures in the anterior chamber of the eye.

anti-metabolite: Drugs like mitomycin-C sometimes used to decrease scarring and increase success of trabeculectomy surgery for glaucoma.

apoptosis: The name for the mode of retinal ganglion cell death in glaucoma, a form of cell suicide in which a protective mechanism from fetal life is reactivated by the disease.

apraclonidine (Iopidine): An alpha adrenergic agonist eye drop

aqueous humor: The fluid filling the front of the eye that is produced at the ciliary body and exits from the trabecular meshwork and the uveoscleral outflow pathway. The balance between how much is made and how much leaves determines the eye pressure.

argon laser trabeculoplasty (ALT or LTP): An outpatient treatment that can lower eye pressure.

asymptomatic: Describes a condition in which the patient does not know it is happening.

B

benzalkonium chloride: a chemical added to many eye drops to keep bacteria from growing in the solution, a preservative, which can cause allergic reactions.

beta adrenergic blocker eye drops: Eye drops that reduce intraocular pressure (IOP) by decreasing the production of aqueous humor through inhibiting beta adrenergic receptors, a part of the unconscious nervous system, includes timolol, carteolol, betaxolol, levobunolol.

betaxolol (Betoptic): A beta blocker eye drop.

Betimol: A beta blocker eye drop.

bifocals: Eyeglasses with lenses that correct both distance and near vision. Many versions have no dividing line and permit continuously changing power of the lens to allow clear vision in middle distances by positioning the head appropriately (called progressive lenses).

bleb: The visible zone on the upper white part of the eye where glaucoma surgery called trabeculectomy has been performed, often slightly elevated and paler than the surrounding tissues.

Bonnet phenomenon: Visual hallucinations caused by substantial vision loss from glaucoma and other eye diseases, due to large areas of missing vision.

brimonidine (Alphagan P): An alpha adrenergic agonist eye drop.

brinzolamide (Azopt): An alpha adrenergic agonist eye drop.

C

carbonic anhydrase inhibitors: Eyedrops or pills that decrease the production of aqueous humor by inhibiting a chemical (enzyme) in the ciliary body.

carteolol (Ocupress): A beta blocker eye drop.

cataract: Haziness or clouding of the lens in the eye that can be removed by surgery.

central corneal thickness (CCT): The thickness of the clear front tissue of the eye, which changes the eye pressure reading when it is thicker or thinner than average.

central vision: The portion of the visual system that does fine, detailed vision.

choroid: The layer of the eye between the sclera and the retina, containing many blood vessels.

choroidal expansion: Thickening of the choroid, which plays a role in causing forms of angle closure and angle closure glaucoma. Sometimes referred to as choroidal detachment.

ciliary body: The part of the eye that makes aqueous humor, found just behind the iris.

ciliodestruction: A laser procedure done in the operating room to lower pressure by decreasing production of aqueous humor.

cones: receptor nerve cells in the retina that capture light and perform detailed vision and color vision.

conjunctiva: the membrane covering the front surface of the eye outside the cornea, like plastic sandwich wrap with blood vessels, that forms the bleb to soak up aqueous humor after trabeculectomy surgery.

continuous wave laser (argon or diode type): Laser used to treat either the angle or the ciliary body to decrease eye pressure.

cornea: The clear front portion of the eye, shaped in a near circle about 12 millimeters in diameter.

corticosteroid: Medicines that are based on normal body hormones, used to decrease inflammation, and often a cause of higher eye pressure when taken as pills, nasal sprays, or inhalers.

D

decibel: The units used in the visual field test that measures how much side vision is lost in glaucoma.

diabetes mellitus: A general body disease of unresponsiveness to or lack of insulin that can lead to a form of secondary glaucoma due to growth of abnormal blood vessels (neovascular glaucoma). Formerly thought to be a contributor to open angle glaucoma, but now known not to be.

diode laser ciliodestruction: A laser procedure done in the operating room to lower pressure by decreasing production of aqueous humor.

dipivefrin (Propine): An alpha adrenergic agonist eye drop.

dorzolamide (Trusopt): A carbonic anhydrase inhibitor eye drop.

dry eye syndrome: Also known as keratitis sicca, a very common cause of stinging, burning, red eyes, treated by use of over the counter artificial tears.

E

edema: A medical term for swelling. When the retina swells in the part that governs reading, it is called macular edema. When the cornea is swollen from high eye pressure, it is corneal edema.

endophthalmitis: Serious infection caused by bacteria, virus or fungus in the inside of the eye.

ethnicity: A preferred term for what is sometimes called race. In this guide, we use the continent from which ancestors of the person came to describe their dominant genetic background, such as, African-derived.

exfoliation syndrome: A disorder that often leads to open angle glaucoma in which cells produce a fibrous white material that accumulates inside the eye and blocks aqueous outflow. Sometimes called pseudoexfoliation.

F

farsightedness: Formally called hyperopia, this form of needing glasses is seen in persons with smaller than average eyes. They can see better far away than up close. A contributing factor in angle closure glaucoma.

filtration surgery: The term used for trabeculectomy, indicating that aqueous humor filters out of the eye through a created opening.

fiber: The long part of a ganglion cell or other neuron that carries its electrical signal on to the next neuron. Also called the axon.

fluorescein angiography: A diagnostic test for abnormality in the retina caused by diseased blood vessels, used in those with neovascular glaucoma.

G

ganglion cells: The nerve cells in the retina of the eye that die in glaucoma, causing its vision loss.

gene: The units of inherited traits made of desoxyribonucleic acid (DNA) and found in the center of most cells. All the genes in a person together are their genome.

gene therapy: Possible new treatments for glaucoma, some called neuroprotection, insert new genes or DNA into cells in the eye, carried there by virus particles that were re-engineered as delivery devices.

glare: A bothersome problem, especially for those with glaucoma, in which too much light hits the eye and, by scattering inside the eye, causes decreased ability to see effectively.

gonioscopy: The examination technique used to see the angle in the front of the eye to distinguish between open angle and angle closure in glaucoma. The lens used is called a gonioscope.

glaucoma: The eye disease in which ganglion cells die in a characteristic pattern, with specific deepening of the optic nerve head structure and particular loss of peripheral visual field. The primary forms are open angle and angle closure glaucoma.

H

hemorrhage: Leakage of blood from blood vessels.

heparin: A medicine given to prevent blood clotting, which must be taken into account when eye surgery is planned.

hyperopia: Farsightedness, in which persons see better far away than up close. A contributing factor in angle closure glaucoma.

I

ICare tonometer: An instrument to measure eye pressure that does not require anesthetic drops to be used first. Helpful in measuring pressure in children and those with unusual corneas.

inflammatory glaucoma: A form of secondary glaucoma caused by inflammation in the eye (uveitis).

intraocular pressure: The difference between the fluid pressure inside the eye and atmospheric pressure outside, produced by the balance between the amount of aqueous humor made by the ciliary body and the amount flowing out of the trabecular meshwork and the uveoscleral outflow pathway.

iridoplasty: a treatment with laser to alter the shape of the iris, used in a condition called plateau iris syndrome.

iridotomy: Also called iridectomy, it is an opening produced in the iris, most often by laser treatment, for angle closure and angle closure glaucoma.

iris: The colored part of the eye whose central opening or pupil allows light into the eye. Muscles in the iris allow the pupil to get bigger in dim light and small in bright light.

Istalol: A beta blocker eye drop.

L

lamina cribrosa: The supporting tissue in the optic nerve head that is impacted by the stress of eye pressure in glaucoma.

laser trabecular surgery: A treatment for glaucoma that involves treating the trabecular meshwork with up to 100 deliveries of laser energy, either argon laser trabeculoplasty or selective laser trabeculoplasty, to improve outflow of aqueous humor and lower eye pressure.

lens: The clear structure shaped like a jelly-bean found behind the iris in the eye that helps to focus images on the retina. When opaque it is called cataract.

levobunolol (Betagan): A beta blocker eye drop to lower eye pressure

low tension glaucoma: A term that is now known to be incorrect, referring to the many persons with open angle glaucoma who never have eye pressure higher than the range found in the population who do not have glaucoma.

Lumigan (bimatoprost): A prostaglandin eye drop to lower eye pressure.

M

malignant glaucoma: A form of angle closure glaucoma that involves collapse of the vitreous humor in the back chamber of the eye.

marijuana: A mixture of plant material that is now illegal in most states that lowers eye pressure when eaten or smoked.

methazolamide (Neptazane): A carbonic anhydrase inhibitor medication used as a pill to lower eye pressure.

mitomycin-C: A medicine placed on the eye at the time of trabeculectomy glaucoma surgery to improve the success at lowering eye pressure.

myopia: Also myopic or near-sighted, the condition where one can see better without glasses up close compared to far away. Myopic eyes are larger than normal and more susceptible to open angle glaucoma.

myocilin: A protein found in the eye that is associated with a rare form of open angle glaucoma when it is mutated or changed by an inherited condition.

N

neodymium:YAG laser: The laser that is most often used to make a hole in the iris (iridotomy) to treat angle closure glaucoma.

neovascular glaucoma: A form of secondary glaucoma that comes from new blood vessels growing in the angle to block outflow of aqueous humor, often associated with diabetes mellitus or blocked blood vessels in the retina.

neuroprotection: A future form of glaucoma treatment in which retinal ganglion cells will live longer due to treatments that are not related to lowering the eye pressure.

normal tension glaucoma: An outmoded term referring to those with open-angle glaucoma who have normal intraocular pressure. Also called low tension glaucoma.

O

ocular hypertension: Refers to an eye that has eye pressure higher than that typically found in the general population. A contributing factor in most forms of glaucoma.

open angle: The space between the iris and the cornea on the interior of the eye, a circular zone running all around the front of the eye, which is open when the iris is not near the cornea, allowing aqueous humor to flow out easily.

open angle glaucoma: The most common form of glaucoma, found in eyes with open angles.

ophthalmologist: A physician and surgeon who specializes in the diagnosis, treatment, and surgery of eye diseases.

ophthalmoscopy: The examination of the inside of the eye, particularly the optic nerve head and nerve fiber layer, during which damage from glaucoma is visible. Performed with bright lights, a binocular viewing instrument (slit lamp) and hand-held lenses by the eye doctor.

optic nerve head: The opening in the back wall of the eye (sclera) that permits fibers of retinal ganglion cells to pass from inside the eye outward to the brain. The location at which fibers are damaged in glaucoma.

optic nerve: The fibers of ganglion cells after they have left the eye, carrying visual images into the brain on the way to the next relay station in the vision system.

optician: A technician who fits and manufactures eyeglasses and contact lenses.

optineurin: Inherited defects in this protein in the eye are linked to some forms of open angle glaucoma in a small number of persons.

optometrist: A specialist who is trained in the diagnosis of eye diseases and is permitted to prescribe eye drops for glaucoma in the United States.

P

pachymetry: A test to measure the thickness of the center of the cornea (central corneal thickness or CCT), useful in estimating the accuracy of eye pressure measurement.

panretinal photocoagulation: A treatment with laser of the interior of the eye (retina) most often done to decrease new blood vessel growth in diabetes, and as an initial treatment for neovascular glaucoma.

perfusion pressure: Blood flowing into the eye is driven by the blood pressure and its entry is resisted by the eye pressure. The difference between blood pressure and eye pressure is the perfusion pressure—if it falls too low, blood does not get into the eye adequately and this is a contributing factor in some glaucoma patients.

perimetry: The formal name for visual field tests that measure loss of side vision in glaucoma.

peripheral anterior synechiae: Places where the iris has permanently stuck to the trabecular meshwork due to angle closure, blocking some of the outflow of aqueous humor and causing eye pressure to be higher.

peripheral vision: The part of what we see that is not directly in the center of our visual world, and the part that is affected during the early and moderate stages of glaucoma.

pigment dispersion: A condition in which the iris rubs on the structures behind it that hold the lens in place, knocking off pigmented tissue that floats in the aqueous humor and lodges in the trabecular meshwork to cause higher eye pressure.

pilocarpine: An eye drop that lowers eye pressure by stimulating the parasympathetic nerve and muscle receptors in the eye.

plateau iris: A condition in which the iris comes close to the trabecular meshwork and seems to block outflow by having a flat, table like shape. When this plateau shape is present but no other problem is present it is called plateau iris configuration. When the eye has repeated attacks of high pressure despite a laser iris hole being made in an eye with this configuration, it is called plateau iris syndrome.

Plavix: A pill medication given to thin the blood and to decrease blood clotting in several general body conditions. Persons using this medication should inform an eye surgeon prior to surgery.

presbyopia: Loss of the ability to see at reading distance that develops in all persons starting at age 45 or so.

preservative: The chemical(s) put in eye drops to keep bacteria from growing in the solutions. Sometimes a cause of allergy to drops.

prostaglandin eyedrops: A group of eye drops commonly used to lower eye pressure in glaucoma.

ptosis: Drooping of the eyelid, caused by age and made worse in some persons by eye surgery. (the "p" is silent).

pupil block: The reason that eye pressure goes high in angle closure eyes. As aqueous humor moves between the iris and lens to get from the back chamber to the front chamber of the eye, it can be blocked, causing the iris to bow forward and leading to closure of the angle.
pupil: The black, circular opening in center of the iris that gets bigger in the dark and smaller in bright light.

R

refractive surgery: Operations most commonly performed with lasers to change the need for eyeglasses. These procedures should be carried out with caution in those with glaucoma.

retina: The innermost layer of the eye wall, that has nerve cells that perform our seeing function. Retinal ganglion cells in this layer are those that die in glaucoma.

risk factor: A feature of a person that contributes to disease, things like age, eye pressure, history of the disease in the family.

S

sclera: The outer wall of the eye, the white part, that determines the amount of stress delivered to ganglion cells in glaucoma. During trabeculectomy glaucoma surgery, a valve-like flap area is created in the sclera to allow aqueous to leak out slowly.

secondary glaucoma: Glaucoma that occurs to an eye due to a second problem in the eye; for example, after a substantial injury.

selective laser trabeculoplasty (SLT): A form of laser treatment to the angle, like argon laser trabeculoplasty (ALT).

side effects: Undesirable results of taking medicine.

slit lamp: The main instrument used by eye doctors to look at the eyes, consisting of a bright light and a viewing set of lenses that look like binoculars.

T

tears: The liquid on the surface of the eye that increases when we cry. Tears come from a gland on the upper, outer part of the tissues around the eye and leave from tubes on the nose side. This is a different fluid from the aqueous or vitreous humor inside the eye and tears do not have anything directly to do with glaucoma. Not having good quality tears is a cause of dry eye, an uncomfortable condition.

threshold: The way in which the visual field test decides how well we see at each of many points that it tests. Formally, threshold is a brightness of the test light that you have a 50:50 chance of seeing against the dim background.

timolol (Timoptic, Istalol): A beta blocker eye drop that lowers eye pressure.

tonometer (tonometry): The instrument (and process) that is used to measure eye pressure.

trabecular meshwork: The part of the angle through which aqueous humor flows out.

trabeculectomy: The most commonly performed surgical operation for glaucoma.

trabeculotomy: The specific operation performed in infants and children for glaucoma. An alternative operation that is similar in children is goniotomy.

travoprost (Travatan Z): A prostaglandin eye drop to lower eye pressure.

tube—shunt: A device consisting of a micro-tube connected to a reservoir that are sewn into the front chamber of the eye and attached outside the eye to allow aqueous to drain out in a surgical procedure.

U

ultrasonic biomicroscopy: An examining method that produces a picture of the inside structures of the eye by using painless sound waves.

unilateral trial: The method in which eye drops are tested for their effect by using them in one eye only for a while. When drops are stopped in one eye to see if they are working, it is a unilateral stop trial.

uveitis: A group of conditions in which there is inflammation inside the eye, sometimes causing a secondary glaucoma.

uveoscleral pathway: A second way that aqueous humor leaves the eye (in addition to the trabecular meshwork). It is a pathway through the space between the sclera and the choroid.

V

vitrectomy: An operation that removes the vitreous humor from the back chamber of the eye, which is needed as the treatment for malignant glaucoma, an unusual form of angle closure.

visual field test: The test used to tell if glaucoma has caused damage to the ability to see, most concentrated in the middle peripheral vision, more formally known as perimetry.

vitreous humor: A gooey substance that fills the back 3/4ths of the eye, and a contributing factor in malignant glaucomaa.

vehicle: The solution in which eye drop medicines for glaucoma are dissolved, including the water in the bottle and chemicals to preserve the drug and keep it effective.

W
warfarin (Coumadin): A drug used to thin the blood, to prevent clotting in a group of general body diseases. Patients taking this medicine should tell their eye doctors before having surgery.

X
Xalatan (latanoprost): A prostaglandin eye drop to lower eye pressure.

Made in the USA
Lexington, KY
08 April 2012